Series editor
Daniel Horton–Szar
BSc (Hons)
United Medical and Dental
Schools of Guy's and
St Thomas's Hospitals
(UMDS),
London

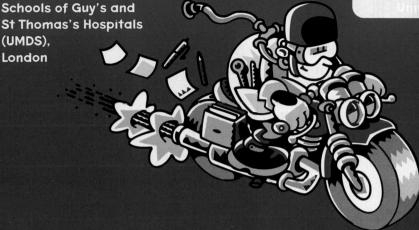

Nervous System and Special Senses

Daniel Lasserson
BA (Hons) Cantab.
United Medical and
Dental Schools of Guy's
and St Thomas's
Hospitals (UMDS),
London

Carolyn Gabriel
BSc (Hons), MBBS, MRCP
Research Fellow in
Neurology,
Guy's Hospital,
London

Basil Sharrack
MD, MRCP, DHMSA
Research Fellow in
Neurology,
Guy's Hospital,
London

£14.95

M Mosby

London • Philadelphia
St Louis • Sydney • Tokyo

Publisher	**Dianne Zack**
Managing Editor	**Louise Crowe**
Development Editors	**Filipa Maia**
	Marion Jowett
Project Manager	**Linda Horrell**
Designer	**Greg Smith**
Layout	**Greg Smith**
Illustration Management	**Daniel Pyne**
Illustrators	**Sandie Hill**
	Debra Woodward
	Joanna Cameron
	Mike Saiz
Cover Design	**Greg Smith**
Production	**Gudrun Hughes**
Index	**Liza Weinkove**

ISBN 0 7234 2989 8

Copyright © Mosby International Ltd, 1998.

Published by Mosby, an imprint of Mosby International Ltd, Lynton House, 7–12 Tavistock Square, London WC1H 9LB, UK.

Printed in Barcelona, Spain, by Grafos S.A. Arte sobre papel, 1998.
Text set in Crash Course–VAG Light; captions set in Crash Course–VAG Thin.

Cataloguing in Publication Data
Catalogue records for this book are available from the British Library and the US Library of Congress.

Preface

Understanding the function of different biological systems is at the heart of medicine and medical exams. This book has been written with the aim of presenting the key facts necessary for a thorough understanding of how the nervous system functions, how it is tested clinically, and how it is affected by disease.

The basic medical science is presented first where the different functional units are described with their clinical relevance. Following this, the neurological history, examination, and methods of investigation are described. In the third section we outline pathology as it relates to clinical practice. In each section we give you the facts needed to understand the core of the subject with plenty of explanatory diagrams and with a focus on areas that have traditionally been difficult to understand.

The author combination of student and doctor brings together experience of undergraduate neuroscience and exams, clinical neurology, and postgraduate research. This balance of authors has enabled us to create a valuable and unique educational tool.

Daniel Lasserson
Carolyn Gabriel
Basil Sharrack

This book offers an innovative approach to the education of medical students combining, in one text, the basic science required to understand the nervous system together with the neurological examination itself.

The first part has been written by a senior medical student and represents the knowledge that a student at the top end of the academic spectrum sees as the essential neuroscience for exam success. The reader will be able to use this part as a revision source or, alternatively, as a useful basis from which to explore the subject further. The essentials necessary to proceed to the clinical part of the medical curriculum are presented.

The second and third parts cover neurological aspects and have been written by neurology registrars. This book is sufficiently comprehensive to allow any medical student to become conversant with the essential knowledge needed to understand how the nervous system functions and how it can become upset in the various disease processes to which it can be subjected.

Anthony Angel
Faculty Advisor

Preface

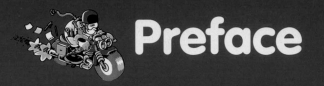

OK, no-one ever said medicine was going to be easy, but the thing is, there are very few parts of this enormous subject that are actually difficult to understand. The problem for most of us is the sheer volume of information that must be absorbed before each round of exams. It's not fun when time is getting short and you realize that: a) you really should have done a bit more work by now; and b) there are large gaps in your lecture notes that you meant to copy up but never quite got round to.

This series has been designed and written by senior medical students and doctors with recent experience of basic medical science exams. We've brought together all the information you need into compact, manageable volumes that integrate basic science with clinical skills. There is a consistent structure and layout across the series, and every title is checked for accuracy by senior faculty members from medical schools across the UK.

I hope this book makes things a little easier!

Danny Horton-Szar
Series Editor (Basic Medical Sciences)

Acknowledgements

Daniel Lasserson would like to thank Professor Angel for his detailed and perceptive comments, Helena Malhomme de la Roche for turning words into pictures, and the staff at Mosby for turning this into a book.

Carolyn Gabriel is currently funded by the British Brain and Spine Foundation.

Basil Sharrack is funded by a grant from Ares-Serono.

Figure Credits
Figures 4.24 and 7.1 (adapted from *Integrated Pharmacology* by Professor C Page, Dr M Curtis, Dr M Sutter, Dr M Walker, and Dr B Hoffman, Mosby International, 1997).

Figures 8.1 and 8.2 (adapted from *Human Histology 2e*, by Dr A Stevens and Professor J Lowe, Mosby, 1997).

Figures 12.3, 11.6, 11.9, 12.7, 12.8, 12.20, 12.24, and 12.25 (courtesy of *Clinical Examination 3e*, by Dr O Epstein, Dr D Perkin, Dr D de Bono, and Dr J Cookson, Mosby International, 1997).

Figures 13.11A, 13.11B, and 13.19 (courtesy of *Imaging Atlas of Human Anatomy 2e*, by Dr J Weir and Dr P Abrahams, Mosby International, 1997).

Contents

Contents

Dedication

To Jane, as it made her summer miserable **DL**

To Isobel, who arrived with the proofs, and to Nick **CG**

To Sawsan, Noor, and Sana **BS**

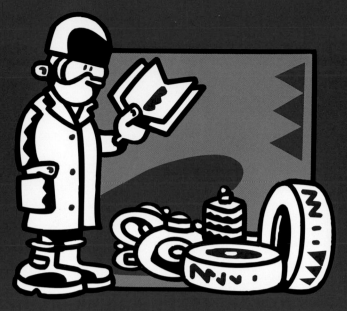

DEVELOPMENT, STRUCTURE, AND FUNCTION

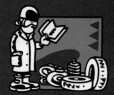

1. Overview of the Nervous System

INTRODUCTION

The nervous system can be divided into three parts:
- The central nervous system processing sensory, motor, and special-sense information, as well as thought, emotion, and regulation of the internal environment.
- The peripheral nervous system providing the sensory and motor innervation to skin, muscle, and bone.
- The autonomic nervous system innervating internal organ systems.

The smallest functional unit in all of these parts is the neuron. In the central nervous system, neurons are surrounded by many other cells with supportive functions. The processing systems of the nervous system are created by communication between neurons. Communication can occur because neurons are excitable cells with the ability to move electrical signals along their length and influence the activity of other neurons through specialized structures called synapses, described more fully in Chapter 2.

Neurons can change physical information into electrical signals. In Chapter 3, we show how the sensory system receives information and transmits it to the brain, and how this information is represented in the brain.

In addition, neurons can influence the activity of other types of excitable cell—smooth and skeletal muscle fibres. In Chapter 4, we describe the control of muscle activity at the different levels of the nervous system (from spinal cord segments to motor cortex) and the strategies of motor planning.

The reticular formation and autonomic nervous system regulate and control the internal environment. We look at these parts in Chapters 5 and 6, and describe how the reticular formation regulates the level of awareness, showing how this can be manipulated to produce general anaesthesia.

Reception and processing of information into the senses of vision, olfaction (smell), and taste are discussed in Chapters 7–9.

The central nervous system is responsible for cognitive functions (Chapter 10). Different thought processes can be localized to different areas of the brain and, to an extent, drug therapy can reverse disordered processing of thought and emotion.

OVERALL DEVELOPMENT OF THE NERVOUS SYSTEM

The fully developed central nervous system is shown in Fig. 1.1. The development of its component parts—the spinal cord, brainstem, and forebrain—follows from the formation of the neural tube by a process called neurulation.

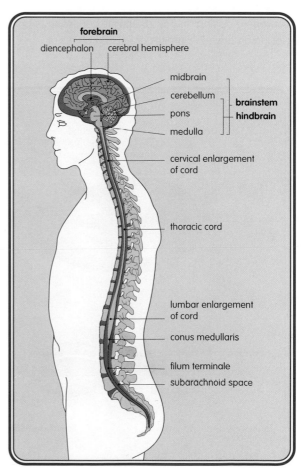

Fig. 1.1 Midsagittal section of the central nervous system *in situ.*

Neurulation

The nervous system develops from a specialized area of embryonic ectoderm called the neural plate. The neural plate forms a longitudinal groove with a ridge on either side.

Neurulation is the process by which the groove fuses at its dorsal extreme to form a hollow tube—the neural tube—and the ridges join up and split off to form the neural crest.

- The neural tube becomes the brain and spinal cord.
- The neural crest cells migrate to form dorsal root ganglion cells, ganglion cells of the sympathetic system, Schwann cells, melanocytes, and musculoskeletal elements of the head and neck.

Neurulation starts on day 22 at roughly halfway along the neural plate (adjacent to the fourth pair of somites), leaving the cranial (head) and caudal (tail) ends open. Neurulation then spreads along the neural groove to close off the tube completely, with the cranial neuropore closing on day 25 and the caudal neuropore closing on day 27. (Somites are paired blocks of mesoderm, segmentally arranged alongside the neural groove of the embryo.) The stages of neurulation are shown in Fig. 1.2.

By the end of development, the segmental arrangement of the nervous system is retained only in the spinal cord.

As the central nervous system develops, an angle forms between the midbrain and forebrain so that the cerebral hemispheres and thalamus are rotated forwards at the top of the brainstem. This rotation explains why the ventral anatomical direction is used to describe both the part of the brain resting on the skull base and the anterior half of the spinal cord.

Embryology of the spinal cord

The spinal cord develops from the part of the neural tube that is caudal to the fourth pair of somites. After neurulation, the lateral walls of the tube (covered by neuroepithelium, which forms the neurons and glia of the cord) thicken, with cells forming two plates on each side, one anterior (basal plate) and one posterior (alar plate). These two plates are separated by a shallow

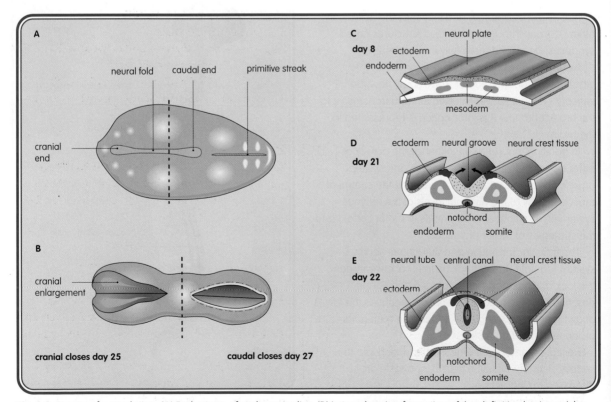

Fig. 1.2 Stages of neurulation. (A) Early stage of embryonic disc. (B) Later, showing formation of the definitive brain vesicles and spinal canal. (C–E) Transverse sections of neural tube taken at different stages of development.

groove—the sulcus limitans. By week 10, the lumen of the neural tube has become a very small central canal.

- The alar plate cells develop into ascending projection neurons and interneurons, which are involved in the sensory pathways and reflex circuits of the cord.
- The basal plate cells differentiate into motor neurons, which are involved with transmission of information out of the cord to muscles, and interneurons. Cells in the thoracic segments of this plate develop into sympathetic preganglionic neurons, whereas cells in the sacral segments develop into parasympathetic preganglionic neurons.

Fig. 1.3 shows the formation and development of the alar and basal plates.

The meninges around the spinal cord develop from mesenchymal tissue surrounding the neural tube, which forms a membrane. The inner layer of this membrane becomes the pia mater, and the outer layer becomes the dura mater.

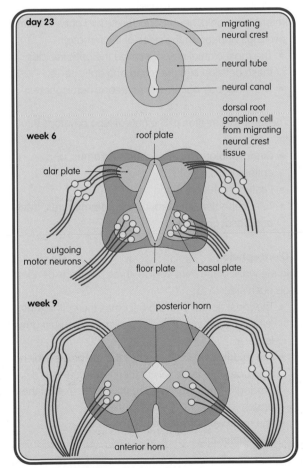

Fig. 1.3 Cross-sections through developing spinal cord.

During development, the spinal column lengthens more than the spinal cord. In the early embryo, the spinal cord runs the length of the column; in neonates (newborn infants), the cord stops at the level of L3; in adults, the cord stops at L1.

Failure of the caudal neuropore to close results in disruption of the lumbar and sacral segments of the cord. Structures that lie superficial to the cord are also involved (e.g. meninges, vertebral arch, paravertebral muscles, and skin), because their development relies upon closure of the neural tube.

Malformations involving the vertebral arch and the cord are called spina bifida.

Embryology of the brain
General arrangement
The brain develops from the part of the neural tube that is cranial to the fourth pair of somites.

When the cranial neuropore closes (by week 4), three vesicles are formed. Fig. 1.4 shows how the three vesicles develop.

Development of the brainstem
The brainstem has the same basic structure as the spinal cord, except that it has to accommodate the large motor and sensory tracts that run between the spinal cord and the brain.

Medulla
The medulla is structured like the spinal cord, with posterior sensory cell groups and anterior motor cell groups. As the medulla flattens out, forming the floor of the fourth ventricle, the posterior (sensory) cell groups move laterally, with some migrating to form the olivary complex.

This means that nuclei dealing with incoming information are found lateral to those sending information out of the medulla (e.g. to skeletal muscle or smooth muscle in the gut, eye, etc.).

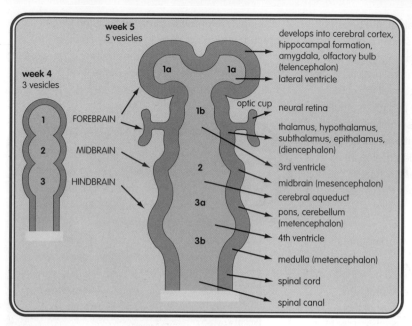

Fig. 1.4 Development of the brain.

Within the figure:

week 5
5 vesicles

week 4
3 vesicles

FOREBRAIN
MIDBRAIN
HINDBRAIN

1a   1a

1b   optic cup

2

3a

3b

develops into cerebral cortex, hippocampal formation, amygdala, olfactory bulb (telencephalon)
lateral ventricle
neural retina
thalamus, hypothalamus, subthalamus, epithalamus, (diencephalon)
3rd ventricle
midbrain (mesencephalon)
cerebral aqueduct
pons, cerebellum (metencephalon)
4th ventricle
medulla (metencephalon)
spinal cord
spinal canal

Fig. 1.5 shows that the cell groups are further subdivided according to whether they innervate body wall structures (somatic nuclei) or organs inside the body cavity (visceral nuclei). Columns of cells are formed with a common pattern that can involve several cranial nerve nuclei.

Pons and cerebellum

The cerebellum develops from the most posterior parts of the alar plates, above the level of the medulla. The cerebellar growths on either side fuse in the midline and migrating cells from the alar plates become the cerebellar cortex.

The pons is formed by the thick band of fibres that connect the frontal lobes, basal ganglia, and thalamus with the cerebellum in a motor processing loop.

Development of the midbrain

The midbrain does not alter much from the basic alar/basal plate structure. The neural canal becomes much narrower forming the aqueduct of the midbrain (also known as the aqueduct of Sylvius).

- Fig. 1.6 shows that the colliculi are formed from migration from the alar plates; colliculi are involved in sensory processing in visual and auditory reflexes.
- The red nucleus and possibly the substantia nigra develop from the basal plates; these are involved in motor processing.

Development of the forebrain

Before the cranial neuropore closes, two pairs of lateral swellings appear on the sides of the forebrain.

- The most cranial pair are called the optic vesicles; these develop into the retina and optic nerve.
- The other pair become the cerebral hemispheres.

The forebrain section of the neural tube develops into the:

- Diencephalon (hypothalamus, thalamus, and epithalamus; Fig. 1.7).
- Posterior pituitary gland.
- Telencephalon (cerebral cortex, commissures, tracts, and basal ganglia).

Diencephalon

In the walls of the third vesicle, three swellings develop on each side:

- The most dorsal swelling becomes the epithalamus (which becomes relatively smaller as the brain grows larger).
- The middle swelling becomes the thalamus (which protrudes into the cavity of the third ventricle, gradually reducing in size relative to the rest of the brain).
- The most ventral swelling becomes the hypothalamus.

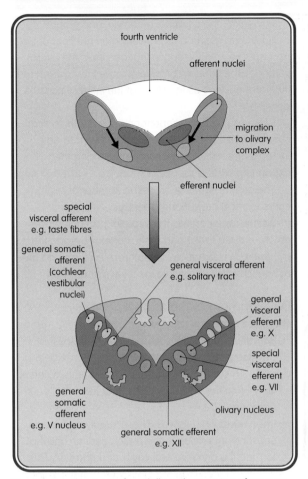

Fig. 1.5 Development of medulla with grouping of sensory and motor nuclei.

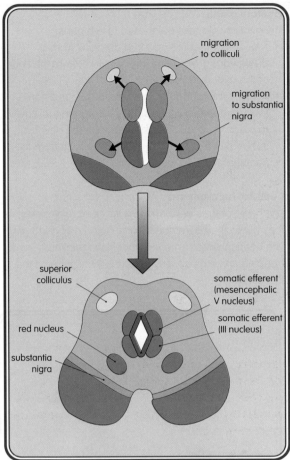

Fig. 1.6 Development of midbrain with grouping of sensory and motor nuclei.

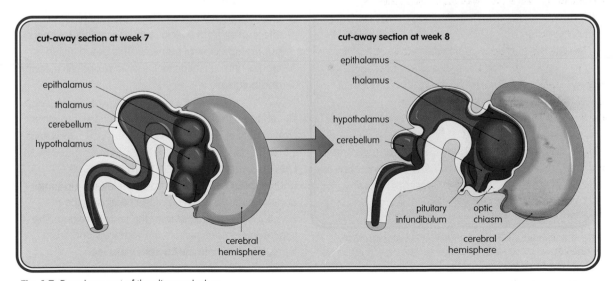

Fig. 1.7 Development of the diencephalon.

Pituitary gland

The pituitary gland is composed of two parts:

- A posterior (neural) part that develops from a downward growth (the infundibulum) from the floor of the hypothalamus.
- An anterior (glandular) part that develops as an inward growth (Rathke's pouch) from the oral cavity towards the brain. It passes through the developing sphenoid bone to reach the downgrowth from the hypothalamus.

Cerebral hemispheres

The hemispheres develop from the cerebral vesicles. As they grow, they cover the diencephalon and midbrain. The hemispheres come together in the midline, trapping some mesenchymal tissue, which forms the falx cerebri.

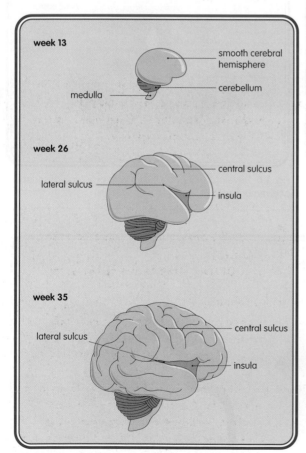

Fig. 1.8 Growth of cortex over the insula and formation of gyri.

In week 6, the caudate, putamen, and globus pallidus start growing as a swelling on the floor of each hemisphere, into the space that becomes the lateral ventricle. The caudate gradually moves away from the lentiform nucleus as the fibres of the internal capsule develop.

Grooves gradually appear on the smooth cortical surface; these become the sulci. The gyri formed increase the surface area, accommodating the expanding cortical tissue.

The commissures grow as the number of corticocortical projections increases.

As the cortex grows, the superior part of it moves down over the lower part of the cortex, covering the putamen. This produces the lateral sulcus and an area of buried cortex (the insula) as shown in Fig. 1.8.

Development of the cranial nerves

There are three groups of cranial nerves:

- Somatic efferents. These innervate muscles that develop from head myotomes (a myotome being part of a somite). This group includes cranial nerves III, IV, VI to the ocular muscles, and XII to the tongue muscles.
- Pharyngeal arch nerves. These supply motor and sensory innervation to the pharyngeal arches that formed the primitive oral cavity and pharynx. This group includes cranial nerves V (from the first arch), VII (second arch), IX (third arch), and X (fused fourth and sixth arches with cranial branch of XI, the accessory nerve).
- Special sensory nerves. These afferent nerves relay information from special-sense receptors to the appropriate central pathway. This group includes cranial nerves I (olfaction), II (vision), and VIII (hearing and balance).

The changing relationship of the arch nerves to other cranial nerves is shown in Fig. 1.9.

Development of the choroid plexuses

Choroid plexuses develop from two layers, pia mater and the ependymal lining of the cavities inside the vesicles, which together form the tela choroidea. The tela choroidea pushes into the ventricles and, from there, develops into the choroid plexuses.

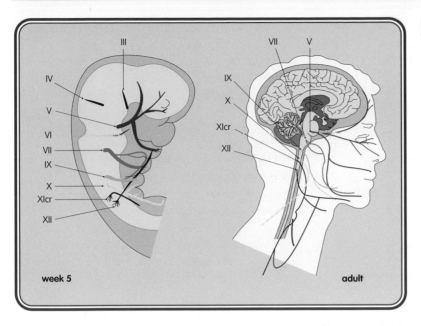

III IV V VI VII IX X XIcr XII

VII V IX X XIcr XII

week 5

adult

Fig. 1.9 Pharyngeal arch nerves in the embryo and adult.

A failure of the cranial neuropore to close can lead to anencephaly. Anencephaly occurs when the cranial vault does not develop, exposing the developing brain. At birth, only the hindbrain structures remain.

- Describe the process of neurulation and the origins of different parts of the nervous system.
- Discuss the structure of the developed spinal cord in terms of the alar and basal plates.
- Summarize the formation of the forebrain, midbrain, and hindbrain.
- Describe the arrangement of the medulla, pons, and midbrain in terms of the alar and basal plates.
- Describe the formation of the thalamus, pituitary gland, basal ganglia, and cortex.
- How does the organization of the cranial nerves relate to their groupings into arch nerves, somatic efferent nerves, and special afferent nerves?
- Give examples of congenital malformations of the spinal cord and brain that occur when the neural tube fails to close.

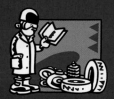

2. Cellular Physiology of the Nervous System

NEURONAL STRUCTURE AND VARIATION

Introduction to organization and function of the central nervous system

The nervous system is essentially very simple. It is formed by networks of neuronal circuits and is best studied if function and structure are related together.

The cells of the nervous system are designed and arranged so that information can be processed, transferred, or transduced. Sensory cells transduce (change) information about the physical state of the environment into electrical signals. These signals are converted into trains of all-or-nothing impulses (action potentials), which are transmitted through axons (see below) to other cells.

Communication between nerve cells occurs at special structures called synapses (Chapter 2). At the synapse, the incoming (presynaptic) information is transferred to the next element in the circuit (postsynaptic), which can be either another nerve cell, a muscle cell, or a gland cell. This transfer occurs either by the release of a specific neurotransmitter (chemical synapse) or by direct transfer of current (electrical synapse).

Processing of information requires that the information is integrated (summed) both in time and from different spatial channels. In some pathways, processing of information occurs by segregation of specific information [e.g. for vision, hearing, somatosensory sensation (touch), pain, etc.]. Processing can be either serial [e.g. in the visual system where patterns of response to light change from the retina (centre/surround spots) to the cortex (centre/surround bars)] or in parallel (e.g. in the visual system where features such as form, motion, and colour are separated and serially processed in three paths, combining to give an integrated image).

The structure of neurons varies reflecting the roles that different neurons have in the processing, transfer, or transduction of information.

Neurons

A typical neuron has the features shown in Fig. 2.1. The dendrites show variable amounts of branching and the more they branch, the more synapses they can form

with the terminal boutons of other cells. The more synapses a neuron forms, the more information it can integrate and process.

The neuron has a large membrane surface area, increasing with the number of dendrites and the length of the axon. A high metabolic rate is required to maintain the integrity of the membrane and to maintain the intracellular ion concentrations by the Na^+/K^+ ATPase pump.

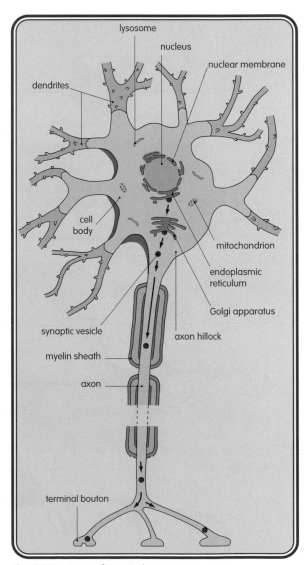

Fig. 2.1 Features of a typical neuron.

The axon is the structure that carries the output of the neuron (the action potential), which is generated at the axon hillock. At the end of the axon are the terminal boutons, which are swellings forming the presynaptic part of a synapse. Variation in these structures results in variation in function, as shown in Fig. 2.2.

Arrangement of neurons

Neurons can be arranged as:
- Layers, e.g. in the cerebral and cerebellar cortices (Fig. 2.3).
- Rods, e.g. motor neurons in the spinal cord.

- Clumps (nuclei), e.g. cranial nerve nuclei in the brainstem.

The differences between projection neurons and interneurons can be listed as follows:
- Projection neurons influence cells located in a different part of the nervous system and so have long axons (often called Golgi type-I neurons), e.g. cortical motor neurons. The long axons often give off small collateral branches that further help to spread information in the central nervous system.

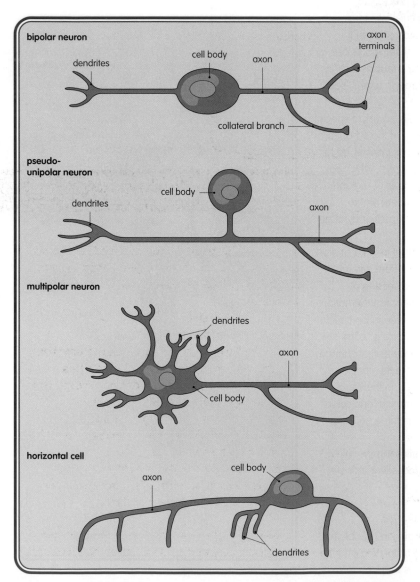

Fig. 2.2 Shapes of unipolar, multipolar, and bipolar neurons, and a horizontal cell.

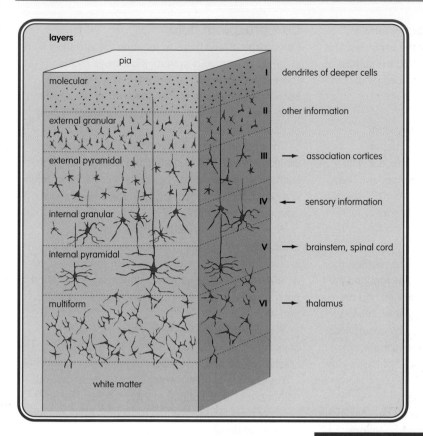

Fig. 2.3 Information flow in the different layers of the cortex.

- Interneurons (termed Golgi type-II neurons) have shorter axons that do not leave their cell group and so provide more opportunities for cells in a group or circuit to communicate with each other. Often the axons give off many collateral branches. This will increase the ability of the cells in the circuit to process information. Humans have a much larger number of these types of neuron compared with their closest evolutionary relatives.

○ **Describe the basic structure of a neuron.**
○ **Describe differences in structure, function, and arrangement of neurons.**

THE CENTRAL NERVOUS SYSTEM ENVIRONMENT

Glial cells

Nerve cell bodies and axons are surrounded by glial cells. There are somewhere between 10 and 50 times more glial cells than nerve cells. Their functions are:

- Physical support.
- Formation of myelin.
- To act as scavenging cells.
- To buffer the external potassium ion concentration.
- To take up and remove chemical transmitters.
- To act as guides (during development) to migrating neurons and direct the growth of axons.
- To induce the formation of tight junctions in endothelial capillary cells, playing a role in the blood–brain barrier.
- There is suggestive evidence that they have a nutritive function for nerve cells, although this has never been conclusively demonstrated.

Glial cells are divided into two classes, microglia and macroglia (astrocytes, oligodendrocytes, and Schwann cells).

Ependymal cells are cuboidal cells that form a single-cell layer around the inside of the ventricles. This layer is continuous with the cells forming the surface of the choroid plexus, which secretes cerebrospinal fluid.

Microglia

Microglia are phagocytic cells that ingest and metabolize foreign material. They are antigen-presenting cells and are capable of interaction with other elements of the adaptive immune system. They are derived from blood monocytes.

Macroglia

Astrocytes

Astrocytes physically support neuronal cell bodies, their axons, and their synapses (Fig. 2.4). They regulate the interstitial fluid potassium ion concentration and are important in preventing the build-up of the inhibitory transmitter γ-aminobutyric acid (GABA) by absorption. They can proliferate to form scar tissue in the event of central nervous system damage.

Oligodendrocytes and Schwann cells

Oligodendrocytes myelinate the axons of neurons in the central nervous system. One oligodendrocyte may myelinate many axons, whereas Schwann cells in the peripheral nervous system are intimately related with, and only myelinate, single axons.

Cerebrospinal fluid

Cerebrospinal fluid helps to regulate the interstitial fluid in the central nervous system. It is formed by the choroid plexus, which is present in all the ventricles. Because the lateral ventricles are largest, the plexus there contributes most to the total cerebrospinal fluid produced.

The choroid plexus is composed of a number of protrusions or villi that arise from a central stalk, which is attached to the wall of the ventricle. Inside each villus is a network of leaky fenestrated capillaries that are adapted for fluid formation.

The cerebrospinal fluid is produced by a combination of capillary filtration and epithelial secretion by carrier-mediated active transport, e.g. for deoxyribonucleosides, folates, vitamins C and B$_6$, and prealbumin (needed for transfer of thyroid hormones and vitamin A).

Blood and cerebrospinal fluid are in osmotic equilibrium because water follows the gradients created by the active transport of solutes.

Cerebrospinal fluid is secreted at a rate of around 0.35 mL/min or about 500 mL/day. Because the total cerebrospinal fluid space (the maximum amount that can be withdrawn by lumbar puncture) is about 150 mL, it must be turned over about three times a day. The intracranial pressure of cerebrospinal fluid is 10–20 cmH$_2$O.

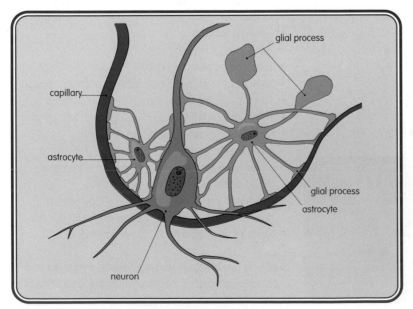

Fig. 2.4 Neurons and glia.

The flow of cerebrospinal fluid is shown in Fig. 2.5.

Outside the ventricles, cerebrospinal fluid flows alongside the deep vascular network within the central nervous system along the perivascular space (Virchow–Robin space). Solutes can diffuse from the interstitial fluid through the pia mater into the perivascular space, as shown in Fig. 2.6.

From the subarachnoid space, cerebrospinal fluid can pass back into the systemic circulation through:

- Arachnoid granulations, which are protrusions of the arachnoid layer into small spaces in the blood drainage system inside the dural folds (e.g. the lateral lacunae of the superior sagittal sinus).
- Spinal nerve roots into the local lymphatic drainage system.
- The cribriform plate into the cervical lymphatics.
- Lumbar cisterns.

This one-way flow of cerebrospinal fluid is a major route for removing potentially harmful brain metabolites.

Hydrocephalus

In the condition of hydrocephalus, there is a blockage in the cerebrospinal fluid drainage route. Consequently, the pressure of cerebrospinal fluid in the ventricles increases as its production is not reduced.

A force is exerted on the brain by the dilating ventricles, which either squeezes the hemispheres against the rigid adult skull or expands the newborn skull. Two forms of hydrocephalus are defined by the site of the blockage.

Non-communicating hydrocephalus occurs when there is a block in the ventricular system, typically by closure of the aqueduct of the midbrain either by congenital malformation or by a tumour.

Conversely, communicating hydrocephalus is caused by a blockage outside the ventricular system in the subarachnoid space.

The differences between cerebrospinal fluid and plasma, both in health and in disease, are shown in Fig. 2.7.

The blood–brain barrier

The blood–brain barrier is formed by a combination of tight junctions between the capillary endothelial cells, the close juxtaposition of the astrocyte end-feet on the capillaries, and the complete absence of fluid phase or carrier-mediated endocytosis as shown by other capillary vessels. These junctions present a very effective barrier to water-soluble substances, but allow some lipid solutes to pass through into the brain, e.g. alcohol.

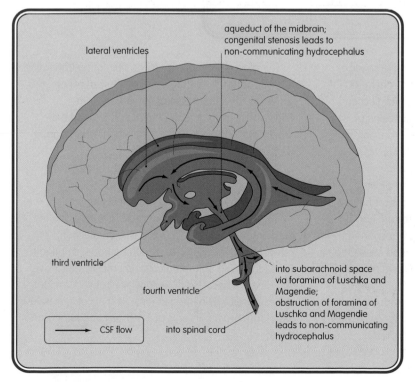

Fig. 2.5 The ventricular system.

lateral ventricles

aqueduct of the midbrain; congenital stenosis leads to non-communicating hydrocephalus

third ventricle

fourth ventricle

CSF flow

into spinal cord

into subarachnoid space via foramina of Luschka and Magendie; obstruction of foramina of Luschka and Magendie leads to non-communicating hydrocephalus

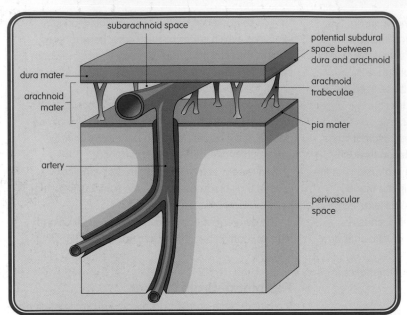

Fig. 2.6 The subarachnoid space.

Fig. 2.7 Cerebrospinal fluid values in health and disease. Values may vary depending on the laboratory (see Fig. 13.10). *The same as 2/3 plasma glucose.

CSF values in health and disease		
	Protein (g/L)	Glucose (mmol/L)
normal CSF	0.15–0.40	2.2–3.3*
CSF in viral meningitis	0.5–1.0	2.2–3.3
CSF in bacterial meningitis	0.50–30	0.0–2.2
CSF in tuberculous meningitis	1.0–6.0	0.0–2.1

Some small hydrophilic molecules have specific membrane transporters—D-glucose is transferred into the cerebrospinal fluid by a stereospecific glucose transporter that simply facilitates the diffusion of glucose. As a result, if plasma glucose concentration drops below 2 mmol/L (e.g. in insulin-induced hypoglycaemia), then glucose will leave the cerebrospinal fluid and go back into the plasma.

There are three separate transporters for neutral (e.g. phenylalanine), acidic (e.g. glutamate) and basic (e.g. arginine) amino acids. L-Dopa is transported by the neutral transporter. Once inside, it can be converted to dopamine and is used to treat Parkinson's disease (Chapter 14).

Ion levels in the plasma can fluctuate abruptly. The blood–brain barrier, together with the Na$^+$/K$^+$ ATPase pumps on the ependymal cells and the high concentration of K$^+$ channels on endothelial cells, help to minimize such changes.

The blood–brain barrier stops circulating transmitters (e.g. noradrenaline) from entering the central nervous system. It also stops central nervous system transmitters from entering the systemic circulation, except at the pituitary where the blood–brain barrier is absent.

The blood–brain barrier is involved in respiratory control, because pH of the cerebrospinal fluid (influenced by HCO$_3^-$ transport) affects respiratory rate.

If the blood–brain barrier breaks down (e.g. after ischaemia, haemorrhage, acidosis, or infection), cerebral oedema can result, with neuronal cell death. For example, in untreated diabetes mellitus, acidosis can develop because of replacement of sodium ions lost in diuresis by hydrogen ions. At a pH of 7 or below, the blood–brain barrier is opened, leading to neuronal death.

Metabolic requirements of the central nervous system

The blood–brain barrier and cerebrospinal fluid provide the fuels and nutrients for cellular metabolism.

The brain requires a continuous blood supply as it cannot store oxygen or glucose and normally does not undergo anaerobic metabolism. To exaggerate the need, it has a high metabolic rate (20% of total body oxygen consumption, 60% of total body glucose consumption), because the Na^+/K^+ ATPase pumps that maintain the osmotic equilibrium across the cell membrane and the resting membrane potential use a great deal of energy.

Blood–brain barrier transport mechanisms can adapt when metabolic requirements change. In starvation, after several days the central nervous system can start to use ketones (acetoacetate and hydroxybutyrate). Initially only 30% of cerebral metabolism is fuelled by ketones, but after prolonged fasting of over 40 days, 70% of cerebral metabolism is based on ketones as fuel.

During development, blood–brain barrier transport of glucose is 30% of the adult level, whereas ketone transport is seven times that of the adult (the energy intake of infants is mainly from fat). Amino-acid transport is higher than adult levels because there is a higher rate of protein synthesis in the developing brain, but this decreases to the adult level over the first 20 years of life.

- What are the functions of glial cells in the support and myelination of central nervous system neurons?
- How is cerebrospinal fluid produced? What is its composition? How does it drain from the ventricles into the subarachnoid space?
- What are the functions of the blood–brain barrier and how do these relate to the metabolic requirements of the brain?

SYNAPTIC TRANSMISSION

Introduction

Input nerve fibres branch repeatedly and end in small swellings called terminal boutons, which form connections (synapses) with the next cells in the circuit.

Synapses are composed of the termination of the incoming (afferent) nerve fibre, a gap and a target cell (neuron, muscle etc.).

Synapses are either chemically or electrically operated (Fig. 2.8) and serve to alter the membrane potential of the postsynaptic cell. For chemically operated synapses, the postsynaptic site contains specific receptor proteins that bind the released chemical.

Types and location of synapses

In the central nervous system, synapses occur on the cell body (axosomatic), on the dendrites (axodendritic), on terminating axons (axoaxonic), and between dendrites (dendrodendritic).

Synapses (Fig. 2.9) are either excitatory (decrease the membrane potential—depolarize—take the cell towards its firing level) or inhibitory (increase the membrane potential—hyperpolarize—take the cell further from its firing level).

Their location can enhance their action. An inhibitory synapse placed close to the axon hillock will more effectively inhibit cell firing than one placed on a dendrite.

The changes in the membrane potential are conducted electrotonically to the cell body, where they are summed.

- Axoaxonic synapses will decrease the release of transmitter from the postsynaptic cell.
- Dendrodendritic synapses possibly cause repetitive activation of a nerve cell to a single input.

Process of transmission

Fig. 2.10 shows the steps between arrival of the action potential, transmitter release and termination of transmitter effect.

Step 1. Action potential arrives at the terminal bouton and opens voltage-gated calcium channels.

Step 2. Calcium ions enter the terminal bouton and allow the vesicles to attach to presynaptic releasing sites. The vesicle membrane then fuses with the presynaptic membrane and the contents are released into the synaptic gap.

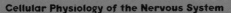

Step 3. The vesicle membrane is then invaginated back into the presynaptic terminal and used to form more vesicles which are filled with transmitter for re-use. This is a dangerous process because it allows extracellular contents to gain access to the interior of the nerve cell (e.g. poliovirus or herpes virus).

Step 4. The transmitter diffuses in the gap to postsynaptic receptors to produce its postsynaptic effect and, in some systems, to presynaptic receptors to regulate transmitter release.

The effect of the chemical transmitter is terminated by one or more of the following mechanisms:

- Enzymatic destruction of the transmitter in the cleft.
- Re-uptake of the transmitter into the terminal bouton.
- Uptake of transmitter into glial cells.
- Diffusion out of the cleft.

Modulation of these mechanisms forms the main basis of central nervous system therapeutics.

Facilitation

If a number of action potentials reach a terminal bouton in a short space of time, then gradually the effect of the transmitter on the postsynaptic cell is enhanced (i.e. either more excitation or more inhibition occurs). This may be because of a build-up of Ca^{2+} within the bouton causing increased exocytosis, as a result of increased Ca^{2+} entry outstripping the removal mechanism.

Fig. 2.8 Comparison of electrical and chemical synapses.

Comparison of electrical and chemical synapses		
Feature	**Electrical**	**Chemical**
cytoplasmic continuity	yes	no
delay	none	0.3–1.5 ms
agent	ion	neurotransmitter
space between cells	2 nm	30–50 nm
direction of signal	one way or both ways	one way
variation in function	either on or off	modifiable activity levels

Fig. 2.9 Types of synapse. Type I, excitatory synapses, depolarize the membrane, whereas Type II, inhibitory synapses, hyperpolarize the membrane.

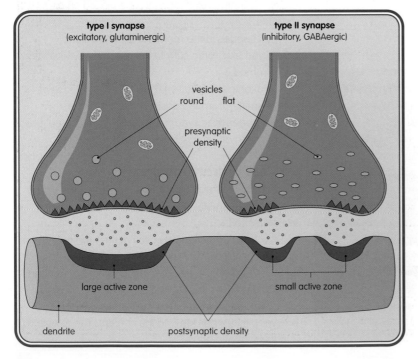

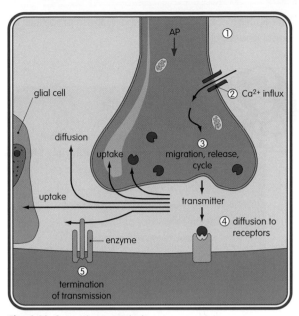

Fig. 2.10 Synaptic transmission.

Neurotransmitters and their receptors

There are four major types of neurotransmitter. An example of the synthesis of each is given in Fig. 2.11.

- Acetylcholine.
- Amines (dopamine, noradrenaline, 5-hydroxytryptamine).
- Amino acids (glutamate, glycine, GABA, aspartate)
- Peptides (opioids, neuropeptide-Y, substance-P, somatostatin).

The effect of a neurotransmitter depends upon the type of receptor that is present at the synapse. Thus one neurotransmitter can have different effects throughout the central nervous system, depending on the receptors it acts upon.

Receptors can be classified according to the second messenger system that they use to alter the membrane potential. Two main classes of receptor are outlined in

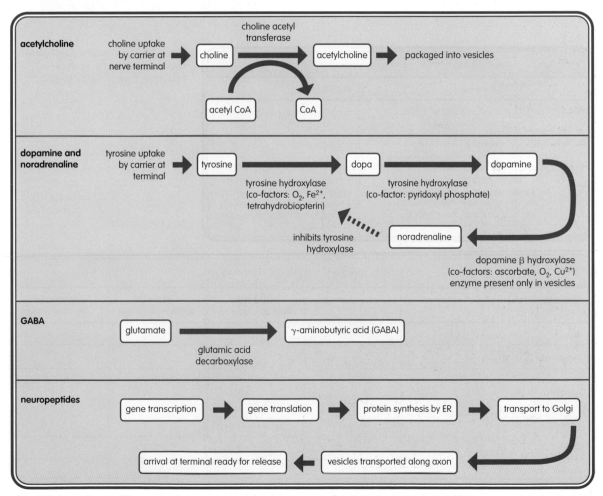

Fig. 2.11 Neurotransmitter synthesis.

Fig. 2.12—the ionotrophic receptor that uses cations and anions as second messengers, and the metabotrophic receptor that is coupled to a G-protein and uses cAMP (cyclic adenosine monophosphate) or IP_3 (inositol 1,4,5-triphosphate) as second messengers that can then have intracellular effects to bring about changes in ion channels to alter the membrane potential.

Receptor diversity for the major neurotransmitters is shown in Fig. 2.13.

Regulation of transmitter synthesis

Transmitter synthesis can be regulated in the short term at the terminal bouton by the intracellular calcium level. If the neuron fires many action potentials, Ca^{2+} will build up at the bouton and increase the activity of Ca^{2+}-dependent protein kinases that can influence the enzymes in the transmitter pathway.

In the longer term, regulation occurs by second messenger action on gene transcription of the

rate-limiting enzyme. Fig. 2.14 shows these processes of dopamine regulation.

- Describe the differences between electrical and chemical synapses, and the importance of different synaptic locations.
- Describe the differences between ionotrophic and metabotrophic receptors.
- Describe the process of synaptic transmission.
- Describe the synthesis of different classes of neurotransmitters.

Structure and function of two main classes of receptor		
	Ionotrophic	**Metabotrophic**
structure	transmembrane ion channel composed of five subunits; binding sites for ligand and modulators outside cell	single transmembrane protein with sites for interaction with ligand outside cell and interaction with G-protein inside cell
functional units	each subunit has four transmembrane domains, and subunits create a charge field to attract either cations or anions; e.g. $ACh\alpha$ subunit attracts Na^+, $GABA_B$ subunit attracts Cl^-	seven transmembrane domains with specific amino-acid residues within domains important for ligand binding; e.g. D_1 receptor has aspartate in domain 3 for dopamine binding

Fig. 2.12 Structure and function of two main classes of receptor: ionotrophic and metabotrophic.

Receptor diversity for the major neurotransmitters					
Transmitter	**Cation channel**	**Anion channel**	**Increased cAMP by G-protein**	**Decreased cAMP by G-protein**	**Increased IP_3 by G-protein**
ACh	nicotinic	$GABA_A$ (Cl^-)		M_2, M_4	M_1, M_3
dopamine			D_1	D_2	
glutamate (channels classified according to experimental agonists)	NMDA (Na^+, K^+, Ca^{2+}), kainate and AMPA (Na^+, K^+)			mGluR2	mGluR1
GABA				$GABA_B$	
opioids				μ, δ	

Fig. 2.13 Receptor diversity for the major neurotransmitters.

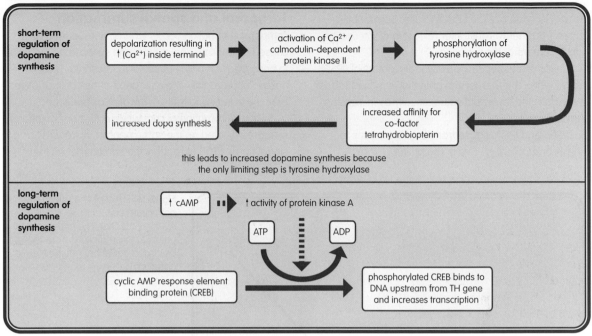

Fig. 2.14 Short- and long-term regulation of dopamine synthesis. (TH, tyrosine hydroxylase.)

EXCITATION AND INHIBITION

Ionic basis of excitatory and inhibitory potentials

Review

To understand excitatory and inhibitory potentials we must quickly review how the resting membrane potential is generated.

If a membrane is freely permeable to a single ion and that ion is found in different concentrations on either side of the membrane, then a voltage across the membrane will be produced. This is what the Nernst equation states and here is calculated for potassium ions:

$$E = \frac{RT}{zF} \log_n \frac{[K_o]}{[K_i]} = -74.8 \text{ mV}$$

and here sodium ions:

$$E = \frac{RT}{zF} \log_n \frac{[Na_o]}{[Na_i]} = 54.3 \text{ mV}$$

R = international gas constant, T = absolute temperature, F = Faraday's constant, z = valency of ion.

The situation is not that simple because membranes are usually permeable to more than one ion and the membranes are not necessarily freely permeable to all the ions.

So we must take different ions and different permeabilities of ions into account when we analyse how the membrane potential is generated, and this can be done with the Goldman equation:

Membrane potential =

$$\frac{RT/F \log_e (P_K[K^+]_{out} + P_{Na}[Na^+]_{out} + \ldots)}{(P_K[K^+]_{in} + P_{Na}[Na^+]_{in} + \ldots)}$$

P is a measure of the permeability to the ion.

This is clearly seen if the external potassium concentration is altered experimentally—the membrane potential changes in Fig. 2.15 fit the predictions of the Goldman equation and not the Nernst equation.

There is a small inward leak of sodium ions in a resting nerve, due to the constant low permeability of the membrane to sodium, and it is counteracted by the Na^+/K^+ ATPase pump. In the pump, ATP breakdown drives the removal of sodium from the nerve against its electrical and chemical gradient in exchange for the entry of potassium.

Excitation and inhibition

An excitatory postsynaptic potential (EPSP) occurs when the membrane potential of the neuron is moved nearer to the threshold for action potential generation, as a result of alteration in the permeability of certain cations, mostly Na^+ and K^+. The signal to alter permeability comes from neurotransmitter release and interaction with receptors at the synapse.

Similarly, an inhibitory postsynaptic potential (IPSP) occurs when the membrane potential is moved further away from the threshold value, usually by increasing permeability to Cl^-.

EPSPs and IPSPs cause transient fluctuations in membrane potential. This is shown in Fig. 2.16.

Temporal and spatial summation

Temporal summation occurs when a number of EPSPs caused by transmission at the same synapse add together to bring the membrane potential to threshold. These EPSPs have to occur rapidly one after another as the fluctuations they cause individually die away after a short time.

Spatial summation occurs when a number of different synapses located on the same neuron all transmit a signal for an EPSP at roughly the same time. All the

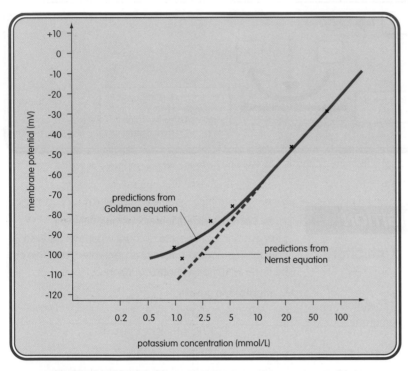

Fig. 2.15 Effect of changing external potassium concentration on the resting potential. The experimental point fit the predictions from the Goldman equation, not the Nernst equation.

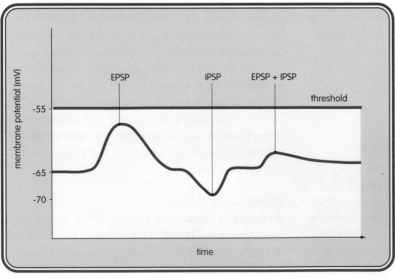

Fig. 2.16 Effects of excitatory postsynaptic potential (EPSP) and inhibitory postsynaptic potential (IPSP) on the membrane potential.

EPSPs can add to bring the membrane potential to threshold.

Generation and propagation of the action potential

The action potential is the result of all synaptic transmissions on a neuron. It is effectively the sum of the EPSPs and IPSPs and they are integrated at the point of action potential generation—the axon hillock.

- The axon hillock has a high concentration of sodium channels and a reduced threshold of action potential generation.
- The action potential is a sudden change in the membrane potential caused by a dramatic increase in the permeability to sodium as shown in Fig. 2.17.

Depolarization opens sodium channels, which results in sodium entry into the axon, causing more depolarization and more open channels and more sodium entry. This will suddenly bring the membrane potential closer to the Nernst potential for sodium (around +50 mV).

The sodium channels quickly shut (inactivate), but from the start of the depolarization potassium channels slowly open. Both these events cause the membrane

potential to swing back to nearer that of the Nernst potential for potassium (around −80 mV).

The membrane briefly becomes more negative (hyperpolarization) than in the resting state as the extra potassium channels that opened during depolarization are slow to close.

The sodium channels will not open again until the membrane is restored to its resting level, no matter how hard they are stimulated. This causes an absolute refractory period.

After the absolute refractory period the sodium channels will only open to greater than normal currents because of the lingering increase in permeability to potassium causing a relative refractory period.

The action potential is propagated along an axon as follows:

- Depolarization occurs in the axon hillock membrane, becoming positive with respect to the resting membrane ahead.
- Current passes across the membrane to the more negative resting region causing the opening of voltage-gated sodium channels. This makes this region positive with respect to both the adjacent part of the axon ahead and the area of the hillock behind.

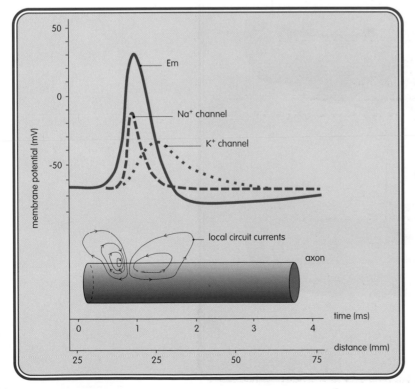

Fig. 2.17 Relationship between opening of ion channels and membrane potential (Em).

- Currents pass forward to the next section of membrane and also back to the hillock but as the hillock is now in a refractory state (absolute or relative) it will not depolarize. Thus the local circuit currents only produce action potentials in membrane areas ahead of the depolarized area.

In myelinated axons, depolarization occurs only at nodes of Ranvier as this is where most of the sodium channels are located and this is the only part of the axon that is in contact with the extracellular fluid. The current therefore travels along the myelinated portion of the axon (i.e. between nodes), only depolarizing the membrane when it reaches a node. This is called 'saltatory' conduction and is shown in Fig. 2.18.

Velocity of action potentials

The factors limiting the movement of the action potential along the axon are:

- Axonal diameter—the larger the diameter, the lower the internal resistance.
- Membrane conductance—if poorly insulated, the axon leaks charge.
- Membrane capacitance—current is used up charging the membrane.

Myelin reduces membrane conductance and reduces membrane capacitance. Less charge is lost through the membrane if the axon is myelinated.

As a rough guide, the velocity of an action potential in a myelinated axon (in metres per second) is six times the diameter (in microns).

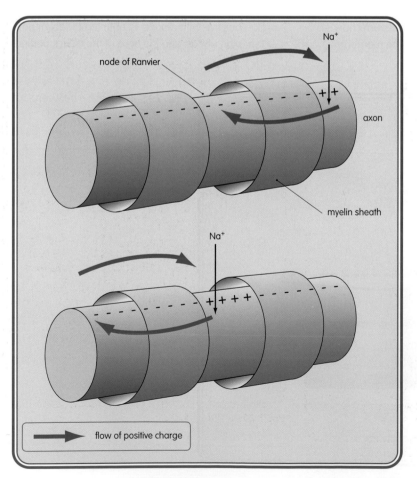

Fig. 2.18 Saltatory conduction in a myelinated axon.

Neural networks

Different sorts of processing require different arrangements of connections in a neuronal circuit. Neurons that form the output from a particular circuit are integrating information from that circuit and sending it elsewhere. An extreme example is the cortical motor neuron that sends its axon in the corticospinal tract. A large number of neuronal contacts converge on the cell; this shows that a number of different circuits govern voluntary movement.

Sensory information coming into the brain needs to go to different areas for processing. Pain, for example, has components of localization, intensity, and unpleasantness, yet only a few receptors send this information to the central nervous system. The neurons in this circuit show a diverging pattern of connections so that similar information can go to different areas that are responsible for different aspects of pain perception.

Fig. 2.19 shows patterns of divergence and convergence. Some circuits show a pattern that is somewhere in between convergence and divergence. Visual information is initially kept separate as it is processed in the central nervous system. This means that when certain neuronal pathways are active, the brain appreciates that information is coming in from a restricted part of three-dimensional space and this increases our perceptual abilities. At higher levels this information is much more integrated so that we consciously perceive a picture rather than a collection of lines and colours in different areas.

At the cellular level, arrangements of inhibitory connections can reduce 'noise'. Noise is neuronal activity that is unconnected with information carried in the circuit (i.e. noise makes the information in a circuit less clear).

There are many patterns of inhibition with different functions:

- Recurrent inhibition is shown in Fig. 2.20 where spinal motor neurons are prevented from firing too often by connections with Renshaw cells.

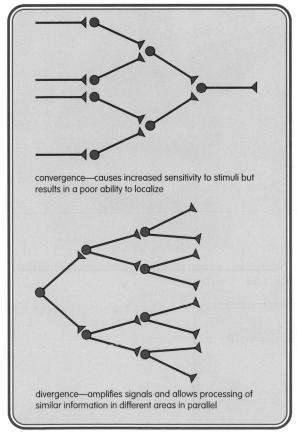

convergence—causes increased sensitivity to stimuli but results in a poor ability to localize

divergence—amplifies signals and allows processing of similar information in different areas in parallel

Fig. 2.19 Comparison of convergent and divergent networks.

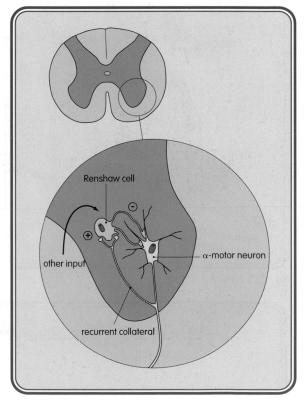

Renshaw cell

other input

α-motor neuron

recurrent collateral

Fig. 2.20 Recurrent inhibition.

- Lateral inhibition is shown in Fig. 2.21 in the retina. Horizontal cells inhibit transmission from photoreceptors that are not illuminated when next to photoreceptors that are illuminated. This means that they create a large difference between the firing pattern of illuminated receptors and non-illuminated receptors. This enables the visual system to be very aware of boundaries between light and dark.

- Presynaptic inhibition is shown in Fig. 2.22. An inhibitory synapse placed on a terminal bouton can reduce the membrane depolarization caused by an incoming action potential, probably by increasing the permeability to Cl^- so that when the inside of the cell becomes more positive with Na^+ current, Cl^- starts to move into the bouton. This will reduce the inward flow of Ca^{2+} and therefore also reduce exocytosis.

- Signalling by disinhibition is shown in Fig. 2.23. As the series of neurons shows, a neuron at the end of a chain can be excited by inhibiting an inhibitory neuron earlier in the chain.

- Inhibition is used in the creation of receptive fields, as shown in Fig. 2.24. The receptive field of a sensory unit can be altered by inhibitory connections with neighbouring sensory units. This can produce a receptive field where the receptor responds to stimulation in one area but is inhibited by stimulation around that area, a so-called 'on' centre and an 'off' surround (e.g. in retinal ganglion cells).

Looking at a higher level, there are networks between large groups of cells as shown in Fig. 2.25. Feedback loops between circuits encourage stable patterns of firing within individual circuits. Parallel pathways occur where different routes are taken to reach the same target groups of cells. This arrangement is useful if one arm of the pathway becomes damaged.

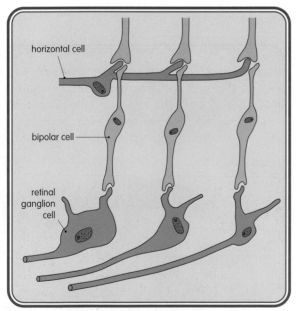

Fig. 2.21 Lateral inhibition.

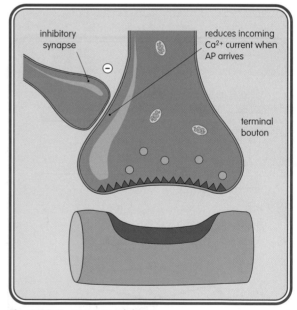

Fig. 2.22 Presynaptic inhibition.

Fig. 2.23 Signalling by disinhibition.

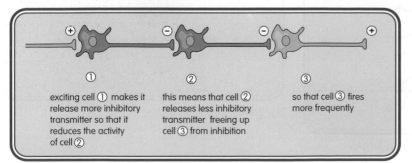

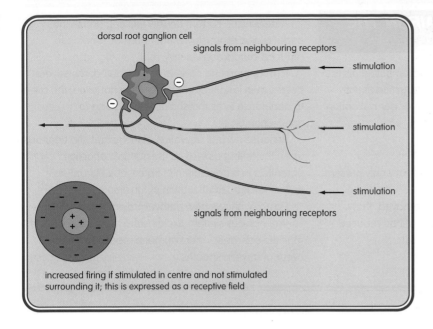

dorsal root ganglion cell

signals from neighbouring receptors

← stimulation

← stimulation

← stimulation

signals from neighbouring receptors

increased firing if stimulated in centre and not stimulated surrounding it; this is expressed as a receptive field

Fig. 2.24 Inhibition and receptive fields.

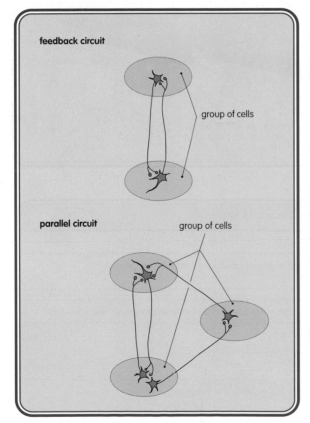

feedback circuit

group of cells

parallel circuit

group of cells

group of cells

Fig. 2.25 Connections between networks.

Connections

Commissural fibres connect neurons in different hemispheres. Association fibres connect neurons in the same hemisphere. Remember that there are vast numbers of connections in the central nervous system and there are many inputs modulating the effects of all connections. This means that even the simple reflex is under many other influences and is not that 'simple'.

- **How is the resting membrane potential generated? How do EPSPs and IPSPs alter the resting potential?**
- **Describe the ionic basis of the action potential in unmyelinated and myelinated axons.**
- **Discuss how patterns of connectivity are designed for different functions. How can inhibition be used in circuits?**

DAMAGE AND REPAIR IN THE NERVOUS SYSTEM

A damaged nerve will not conduct action potentials to its terminal boutons. This block of conduction usually occurs either after section of the axon or demyelination of the axon.

The effect of demyelination

In myelinated axons, sodium channels are only present at the nodal regions.

Fig. 2.26 shows that if myelin is removed, the current density at the nodal regions will be reduced because current will exit across the bare membrane.

A decreased current density will depolarize the nodal region more slowly than normal, leading to reduced conduction velocity.

If more than one node is demyelinated, the severe decrease in longitudinal current may not allow the axon to depolarize to its threshold level, leading to conduction block.

Because normal activation of the target site depends upon the timing as well as the number of action potentials in a population of fibres, any disruption in timing will lead to disruption of function.

Fig. 2.27 shows how demyelination of axons in the central nervous system explains the clinical features of multiple sclerosis, where immune mediated attacks occur on myelin sheaths.

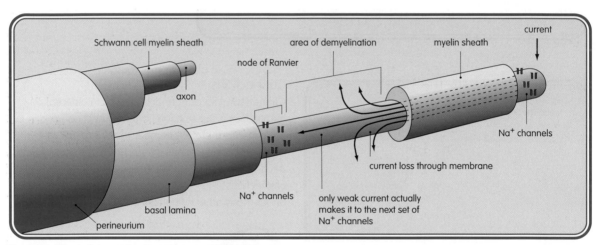

Fig. 2.26 Effect of demyelination on current flow in an axon.

Pathophysiology of multiple sclerosis symptoms	
Symptoms	**Cellular explanation**
blindness, numbness, weakness, paralysis	Block in conduction of action potential caused by dissipation of current after demyelination
paraesthesia (tingling)	Extracellular potassium builds up at sites of demyelination as channels exposed that leak potassium. This raises membrane potential to threshold and action potential generated spontaneously (Nernst equation)
remission of symptoms	Caused by: (A) remyelination by oligodendrocytes (B) use of alternative neural pathways (C) new sodium channels produced
relapse	(A) extension of existing lesion with exposure of membrane with few sodium channels (B) new lesion site
Lhermitte's sign (feeling of electric shock in limbs upon stretching)	Lesions often form in areas of CNS that are constantly being moved, such as the part of the spinal cord in the region of the cervical vertebrae. When lesioned axons are stretched they generate impulses. (A similar problem occurs in the optic nerve and flashes are seen at night when there is much less light to mask the effect of these spontaneous impulses.)

Fig. 2.27 Pathophysiology of multiple sclerosis symptoms.

Responses of peripheral axons to different types of trauma

Fig. 2.26 shows the relationship between a peripheral axon, its associated Schwann cells and thin connective-tissue covering—the basal lamina—which forms a continuous tube containing the axon–Schwann cells complex.

Fig. 2.28 shows that after trauma the main factors influencing restoration of function are the integrity of the axon itself, the integrity of the basal lamina and the length of time needed for regrowth to the site of innervation (i.e. distal muscles may atrophy completely before a nerve sectioned far away grows and reaches them).

Responses of the central nervous system to damage

The central nervous system is hostile to axonal regrowth. Neurons will not grow through glial scars and inhibitory molecules, associated with oligodendrocytes, cause a collapse of the growing tip of the axon.

As a potential therapy, cells secreting antibodies to the inhibitory molecules could be inserted locally in the tissue protecting the growth cone from inhibitory signals. Or, in the case of spinal-cord injury, a piece of peripheral nerve could be inserted above and below the transection to provide a growth-friendly bridge across the gap.

Effects of peripheral nerve injury				
	Compression	Crush	Severed nerve	Severed limb
axon	intact	discontinuous	discontinuous	discontinuous
basal lamina	intact	intact	discontinuous	discontinuous
regrowth possibilities	no regrowth needed, full remyelination within a few weeks	trophic factors released by distal part of axon, and proximal axon (still attached to cell body) regrows at 1 mm/day	trophic factors released by distal part of axon, but can grow into wrong basal lamina, previously occupied by nerve with different function	no distal part of axon present; nerve forms a neuroma
restoration of function	complete	dependent on length of axonal growth needed for reinnervation	four possibilities: 1. grows into original basal lamina 2. grows into basal lamina of same modality—altered function 3. grows into basal lamina of different modality—no function 4. forms neuroma—no function	no function; disturbed sensation and chronic/ transient pain

Fig. 2.28 Effects of peripheral nerve injury.

- What is the effect of demyelination on the conduction of action potentials?
- Relate the symptoms of multiple sclerosis to the processes of damage and repair.
- Name the common types of peripheral nerve injury and the cellular processes of repair that govern restoration of function.
- Describe possible ways to encourage central nervous system repair.

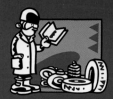

3. The Somatosensory System

THE SPINAL CORD AND SPINAL TRACTS

Spinal cord

The spinal cord is a segmentally organized tube with a central cellular area surrounded by nerve-fibre tracts. The tracts carry information to and from structures above the cord and also to and from other segments in the cord.

Fig. 3.1 shows the relationship between the spinal cord, its coverings, and its bony housing in the vertebral column. As seen in Chapter 1, the cord ends at vertebral body level L1/L2 and so a lumbar puncture needle can be inserted into the subarachnoid space below this level (e.g. L3/L4) without damaging the cord.

Cells

Fig. 3.2 shows that the cells in the grey matter can be divided up as a series of layers in the dorsal horn and as a series of columns in the ventral horn. These layers and columns are known as Rexed's laminae (numbered I–X) and are based on groupings of similarly shaped cell bodies.

The dorsal horn layers are involved in sensory pathways and are the target sites for some sensory afferent nerves, particularly for pain, temperature, and crude touch.

The ventral columns are made up of pools of motor neurons innervating skeletal muscle. Medial motor columns supply proximal muscles and lateral motor columns supply distal muscles.

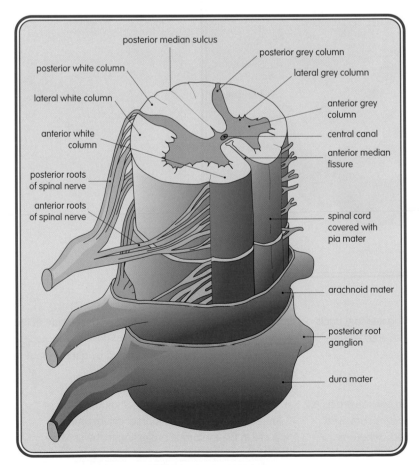

Fig. 3.1 Spinal cord above the level L1. Coverings of dura mater, arachnoid mater, and pia mater are shown.

posterior median sulcus

posterior grey column

posterior white column

lateral grey column

lateral white column

anterior grey column

anterior white column

central canal

anterior median fissure

posterior roots of spinal nerve

anterior roots of spinal nerve

spinal cord covered with pia mater

arachnoid mater

posterior root ganglion

dura mater

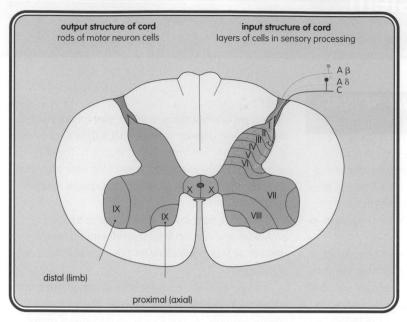

Fig. 3.2 Rexed's laminae (afferent fibres show examples of termination patterns).

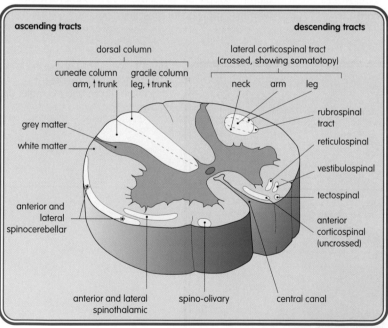

Fig. 3.3 White matter tracts.

Tracts

As a general rule, in the white matter the sensory tracts run in the periphery and motor tracts occupy a more central position, as seen in Fig. 3.3.

Ascending

The major difference between the main sensory tracts is that fine information (dorsal column tract) is conveyed up the cord on the same side as it enters, whereas pain, temperature, and crude touch (spinothalamic tract) are conveyed upwards on the opposite side of the cord.

The sensory tracts are constructed by a three-neuron pathway:
- from the dorsal root ganglion cell to
- a cell in the dorsal horn (spinothalamic tract) or dorsal column nucleus (dorsal column tract) to
- a cell in the thalamus projecting to the sensory cortex.

The sensory tracts are both arranged segmentally, i.e. fibres from the same segment run upwards together in the tract.

The spinocerebellar tract (Fig. 3.4) can be divided into two tracts:

- The anterior spinocerebellar tract begins with cell bodies in lamina VII, which pass axons across to the other side of their segment then up to the cerebellum. This tract sends information about interneuron activity.

- The lateral spinocerebellar tract begins with cell bodies that lie in a column running from T1 to L2. Fibres from dorsal root ganglion cells innervating joints, muscles, and skin synapse with the cells in this column either by travelling up the dorsal column (if they come from below L2) or by directly synapsing when they enter the cord. This tract conveys information about body movement.

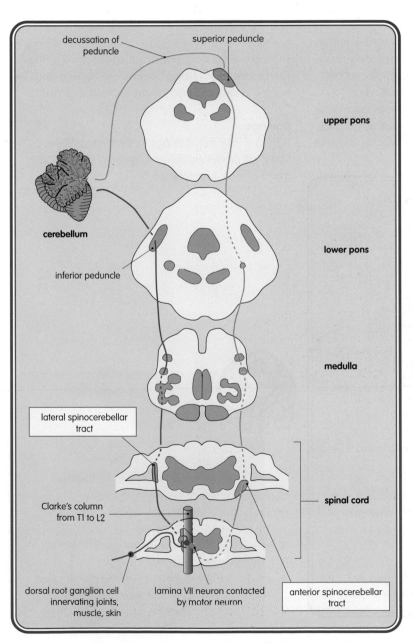

Fig. 3.4 The spinocerebellar tracts.

decussation of peduncle

superior peduncle

upper pons

cerebellum

lower pons

inferior peduncle

medulla

lateral spinocerebellar tract

spinal cord

Clarke's column from T1 to L2

dorsal root ganglion cell innervating joints, muscle, skin

lamina VII neuron contacted by motor neuron

anterior spinocerebellar tract

Descending

The corticospinal tract is the major controller of skeletal muscle activity. It has two branches: the crossed lateral tract controls the precision movements of the limbs (innervating lateral motor neuron pools) and the uncrossed anterior tract controls the less precise movements of the trunk (innervating medial motor neuron pools).

It is organized somatotopically, i.e. fibres innervating motor neuron pools controlling muscle groups run down together in the tract.

The other descending tracts have a crude control of movement.

The tectospinal tract controls head and neck posture. The tract begins with cells in the superior colliculus and their axons cross the midline in the midbrain, but only go as far as motor neurons in the cervical cord.

The vestibulospinal tract acts with the tectospinal to keep the head balanced on the shoulders as the body moves through space and to turn the head in response to sensory stimuli.

The reticulospinal tract (Fig. 3.5) controls posture and helps in the control of crude imprecise movements. The reticular formation is a term used to describe a diffuse network of cells in the brainstem that receives information from a large part of the central nervous system and is involved in the control of many of the body's automatic processes. There are two tracts of note:

- The pontine reticulospinal tract projects to motor neurons innervating axial muscles (in control of trunk posture).
- The medullary reticulospinal tract projects to motor neurons innervating distal muscles (in control of antigravity muscles).

The rubrospinal tract functions are subsumed by the corticospinal tract. Fibres from the red nucleus cross the midline in the pons and join the corticospinal tract.

Damage

Fig. 3.6 shows that damage to the cord at different levels will produce different degrees of deficit in both motor and sensory function.

Fig. 3.5 The reticulospinal tract.

- Give an outline of the function of the spinal cord.
- Discuss the inputs to and outputs from the laminae of the grey matter in relation to the scope for sensory modulation by interneurons.
- Describe the arrangement of the tracts within the white matter of the cord and the arrangement within the tracts.

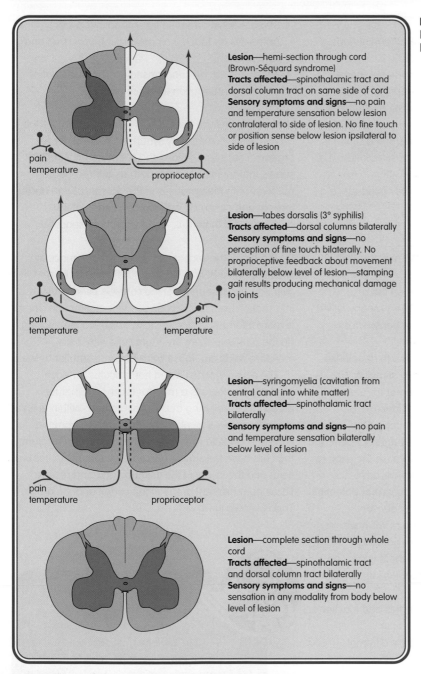

Lesion—hemi-section through cord (Brown-Séquard syndrome)
Tracts affected—spinothalamic tract and dorsal column tract on same side of cord
Sensory symptoms and signs—no pain and temperature sensation below lesion contralateral to side of lesion. No fine touch or position sense below lesion ipsilateral to side of lesion

Lesion—tabes dorsalis (3° syphilis)
Tracts affected—dorsal columns bilaterally
Sensory symptoms and signs—no perception of fine touch bilaterally. No proprioceptive feedback about movement bilaterally below level of lesion—stamping gait results producing mechanical damage to joints

Lesion—syringomyelia (cavitation from central canal into white matter)
Tracts affected—spinothalamic tract bilaterally
Sensory symptoms and signs—no pain and temperature sensation bilaterally below level of lesion

Lesion—complete section through whole cord
Tracts affected—spinothalamic tract and dorsal column tract bilaterally
Sensory symptoms and signs—no sensation in any modality from body below level of lesion

Fig. 3.6 Effects of spinal cord lesions in different areas. Area of lesion is shaded.

SOMATOSENSATION AND THE SENSORY CORTEX

Sensation

If the skin is explored with a stiff nylon bristle then four sensations are reported by humans—touch, heat, cold, and pain.

This can be extended in animal studies to show that individual receptors from the skin respond to touch, pressure, cold, heat, and mechanical nociceptive (pain), thermal nociceptive, and polymodal nociceptive stimuli—called modalities.

In humans, no matter how a receptor is activated (electrically or electromagnetically), the subjective sensation reported is always that of its modality.

This has led to the concept of modality-specific channels that convey information of one modality from the skin to the sensory receiving area.

Receptors

Receptors are formed by the peripheral terminations of the axons of dorsal root ganglion cells.

Identified cutaneous receptors include free nerve endings (pain, thermal, touch, and pressure) or in association with different connective-tissue structures (e.g. pacinian corpuscles, Fig. 3.7)

Receptors signal different properties of the stimulus:

- Tonic receptors signal the degree of stimulation, e.g. Ruffini's corpuscle.
- Phasic receptors signal stimulus rate of change, e.g. Meissner's corpuscle.
- Transient receptors signal the rate of rate of change, e.g. pacinian corpuscle.
- Tonic and phasic receptors, e.g. thermoreceptors.

The different signalling depends either on the linkage of the receptor to its incident energy or on a property called adaptation (i.e. a decline in receptor responsiveness even though the stimulus is still present).

The receptor membrane is influenced to depolarize (the generator potential) by its modality stimulus. This causes a current to flow from the receptor to its axon. If sufficient, this causes the axon to depolarize to its threshold level and produce an action potential. Because the axon will recover after its refractory period, a long-lasting generator potential will cause the axon to fire a train of impulses. Their frequency will be proportional to the magnitude of the generator potential.

To accommodate the wide range of sensory experience, different unimodal receptors will have different thresholds and the generator potential behaves as a power function (so that there is a logarithmic relationship between stimulus intensity and perceived sensation).

Fig. 3.7 shows the structure, properties and functions of cutaneous receptors.

Fig. 3.8 shows different fibre types for different modalities and their conduction speeds and axonal diameters.

The dorsal column pathway

This pathway carries most of the information from the body surface to the contralateral primary sensory cortex. There is a distorted representation of the body in the sensory cortex (the sensory homunculus) and one of the functions of the dorsal column pathway is to reorganize the input from a dermatomic structure to a homuncular structure. This pathway :

- Segregates information into modality-specific pathways for touch, hair movement, pressure, and joint rotation.
- Has feedback mechanisms to gate the amount of incoming information to the cortex.

These functions are carried out in the areas where the pathway is interrupted by synapses, to allow for re-organization, segregation, and suppression. Fig. 3.9 shows the dorsal column system as a three-neuron pathway with the synapses in the dorsal column nuclei (gracile and cuneate), the ventroposterior lateral nucleus of the thalamus, and the primary sensory cortex.

The site of the sensory cortex and its homuncular structure are shown in Fig. 3.10. The homunculus is distorted because more of the cortex is used to process information from body areas used for exploration. There is more information from distal areas because, moving up the pathway, there are more cells with distal receptive fields and those fields become smaller as well.

The sensory cortex has a homunculus for each modality (i.e. there is a map for touch, another for pressure etc., all lying next to each other). Within each modality, there is a columnar organization from the cortical surface to the white matter. Within each column, the cells have the similar response properties (receptive field) and the layers in the column send and receive fibres from different areas of the cortex and thalamus. This is shown in Fig. 3.11.

○ **Discuss the structure and properties of receptors of different modalities and how they code signals.**
○ **What are the variations in sensory fibre type?**
○ **Summarize the arrangement of the dorsal column pathway. How can it rearrange information?**
○ **Describe the functional arrangement of the sensory cortex.**

Fig. 3.7 Structural properties of cutaneous receptors.

Meissner's corpuscle

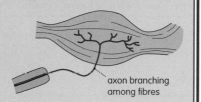

axon winding

location—dermal papillae in glabrous skin (palms and soles of feet)
stimulus—touch
adaptation—rapidlo
threshold—low
modality and function—mechanoreceptor signalling sudden light touch

Ruffini's corpuscle

axon branching among fibres

location—dermis of skin
stimulus—stretch
adaptation—slow
threshold—low
modality and function—mechanoreceptor signalling state of stretch of skin

Merkel's disc

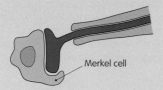

Merkel cell

location—basal layer of cells of epidermis in fingers, lips, genitals
stimulus—pressure
adaptation—slow
threshold—low
modality and function—mechanoreceptor signalling low-intensity constant pressure

Pacinian corpuscle

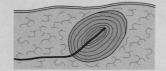

location—junction between dermis and epidermis, vessel walls, joint capsules
stimulus—indentation of skin
adaptation—very rapid
threshold—low
modality and function—mechanoreceptor signalling the start of indentation of the skin

Pain receptor, polymodal pain receptor, and thermoreceptor

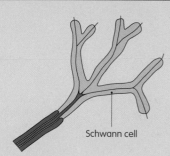

Schwann cell

Pain receptor
location—nerve endings lie free within skin
stimulus—high mechanical force (cuts, stretch)
adaptation—none
threshold—very high
modality and function—nociceptor functioning as a high-threshold mechanoreceptor

Polymodal pain receptor
location—nerve endings lie free within skin
stimulus—high force, heat (>40°C), chemicals
adaptation—none
threshold—variable as can be lowered, e.g. in inflammation
modality and function—nociceptor signalling state of impending tissue damage

Thermoreceptor
location—nerve endings lie free within skin
stimulus—changes in temperature of skin locally
adaptation—rapid
threshold—low (0.2°C rise causes large increase in action potential frequency)
modality and function—thermoreceptor signalling changes rather than absolute temperature

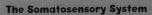

Sensory afferent fibres				
Class	Modality	Axonal diameter (µm)	Conduction speed (m/s)	Pattern of termination in laminae of cord
myelinated				
Aα	proprioceptors from muscles, tendons	20	120	III, IV, V
Aβ	mechanoreceptors from skin	10	60	III, IV, V
Aδ	nociceptor, cold thermoreceptor	2.5	15	I, II, V
unmyelinated				
C	nociceptor, heat thermoreceptor	<1	<1	I, II

Fig. 3.8 Sensory afferent fibres.

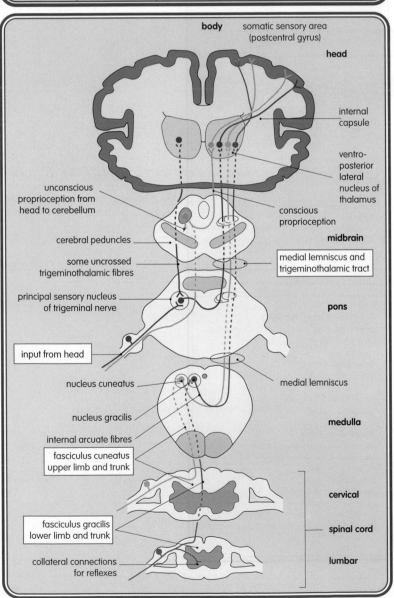

Fig. 3.9 The dorsal column pathway showing pathways for touch and conscious proprioreception. The system is a three-neuron pathway: fine touch from the lumbar and lower thoracic regions, the upper thoracic and cervical regions, and the head; and proprioception from the head.

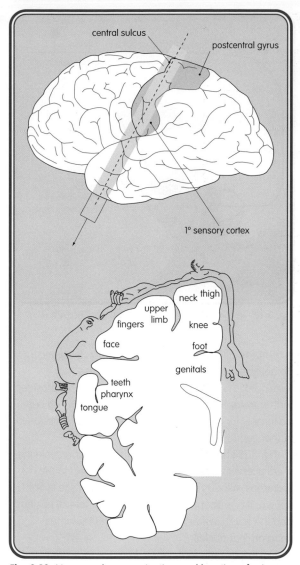

Fig. 3.10 Homuncular organization and location of primary sensory cortex.

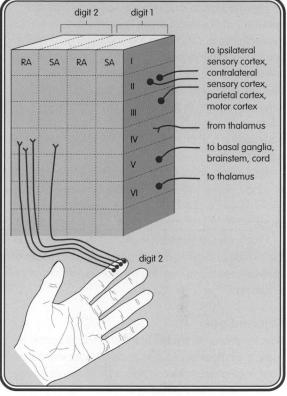

Fig. 3.11 Columnar organization of primary sensory cortex. (RA, rapidly adapting; SA, slowly adapting.)

NOCICEPTION AND THE PERCEPTION OF PAIN

This section deals with the mechanisms and regulation of acute pain (the type of pain that tells us that tissue damage has suddenly occurred). The mechanisms of chronic pain involve distortions in the acute pain pathways.

Nociception

Nociception is the sensory process detecting overt or impending tissue damage. Pain is the perception of irritating, sore, stinging, throbbing, or painful sensations arising from the body.

Although nociceptors do not show adaptation (i.e. they fire continuously to tissue damage), pain sensation may come and go and pain may be felt in the absence of nociceptor discharge.

Nociceptor afferent nerves release not only the excitatory transmitter glutamate (as do all sensory afferent nerves) but also substance-P. This causes a very long-lasting excitatory postsynaptic potential and helps sustain the effect of noxious stimuli.

39

Hyperalgesia is the phenomenon of increased sensitivity of damaged areas to painful stimuli. Primary hyperalgesia occurs within the damaged area and secondary hyperalgesia occurs in undamaged tissues surrounding this area. After damage, blood vessels become leaky and the damaged tissue cells release a variety of chemicals that give a local response—inflammation (e.g. histamine, which directly excites nociceptors, and prostaglandin, which sensitizes nociceptors).

Pain is somehow related to itch. Itch is mediated by Aδ and C fibres; people born without a sense of pain show no sense of itch, but itch is unaltered by opiate drugs.

Processing of nociceptive afferent nerves begins in the circuits in the dorsal horn and a certain amount of control is exercised over the firing of spinothalamic cells in lamina I.

Referred pain

Pain from internal organs (viscera) is felt as pain in a more superficial region of the body. Nociceptor fibres from viscera and from cutaneous structures converge on the same pain pathway (i.e. spinothalamic cells). The central nervous system can make no distinction between superficial pain and deep pain and consequently interprets all pain as superficial. For example:

- Pain of myocardial infarction is felt centrally just behind the sternum, radiating down the left arm and up the root of the neck into the jaw.
- Inflammation affecting the diaphragm is felt in the tip of the shoulder (phrenic nerve root values C3–C5).

Spinothalamic tract and pain signals

In addition to pain, the spinothalamic tract also carries crude touch and thermal information. Pain information is also carried in the spinoreticular and spinomesencephalic tracts.

Noxious and thermal information is carried into the dorsal horn by quicker myelinated Aδ fibres (conveying sharp, stabbing pain) and slower unmyelinated C fibres (conveying dull, nagging pain).

Fig. 3.12 shows that Aδ fibres terminate in laminae I, IV, and V. Cells from these laminae cross over to the opposite side of the cord and ascend in the anterolateral white matter, forming the spinothalamic tract.

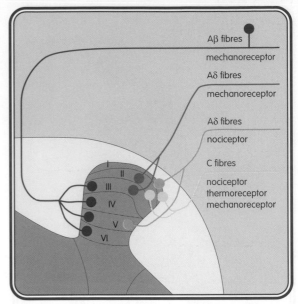

Fig. 3.12 Termination of nociceptive afferent nerves.

C fibres influence the firing of the spinothalamic dorsal horn cells via interneurons, because they terminate in a different lamina—lamina II. This provides further synaptic steps in the pain pathway, which can be targets for modulation of pain signal transmission by higher centres.

Fig. 3.13 shows that the spinothalamic fibres join the medial lemniscus in the medulla and project to the thalamus. Although their exact termination site is not known, it is probably the ventroposterior lateral nucleus and the nuclei inside the laminae in the thalamus (intralaminar nuclei).

Nociceptive afferent nerves from the face are carried in the trigeminal nerve and spinal tract of the trigeminal nerve to the spinal trigeminal nucleus (which takes over the function of dorsal horn laminae I and II). The efferent fibres from the spinal nucleus of V cross over to the other side of the medulla and pass up to the thalamus.

Regulation of pain
Peripheral regulation

Pain can be regulated by sensory input—it can be reduced by activity in low-threshold mechanoreceptors, as their afferent nerves inhibit spinothalamic cell discharge (Fig. 3.12) This has a clinical correlate in the use of transcutaneous electrical nerve stimulation (TENS) to activate large-diameter fibres in some kinds of chronic, intractable pain states.

Central regulation

Pain can sometimes be suppressed by 'willing it to go away'. A possible correlate for this is that there are regions in the central nervous system that have been implicated in pain suppression (Fig. 3.14).

Electrical stimulation of the periaqueductal grey matter in the midbrain causes profound analgesia. This area receives information from higher structures processing emotional states and projects to the midline reticular and raphe nuclei, which in turn project to the dorsal horns.

Two other parts of the reticular formation—the nucleus reticularis paragigantocellularis and the locus coeruleus—are also implicated in modulating nociceptive neuronal activity in the dorsal horns.

Opiates are thought to produce their antinociceptive action by activating these central regulating structures.

Some of these regions contain endogenous opioid peptides, although pain modulation also involves 5-hydroxytryptamine (5-HT) from the raphe nuclei and noradrenaline from the locus ceruleus.

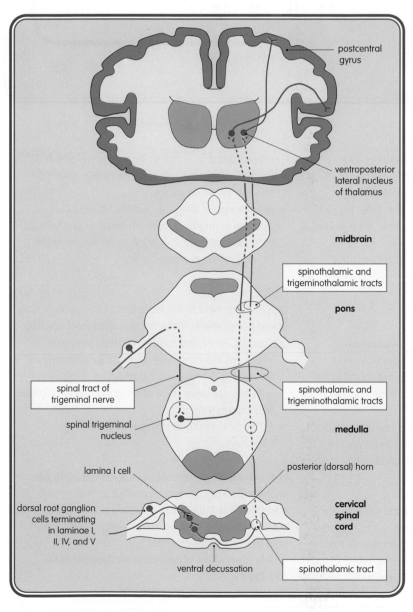

Fig. 3.13 The spinothalamic tract.

postcentral gyrus

ventroposterior lateral nucleus of thalamus

midbrain

spinothalamic and trigeminothalamic tracts

pons

spinal tract of trigeminal nerve

spinothalamic and trigeminothalamic tracts

spinal trigeminal nucleus

medulla

lamina I cell

posterior (dorsal) horn

dorsal root ganglion cells terminating in laminae I, II, IV, and V

cervical spinal cord

ventral decussation

spinothalamic tract

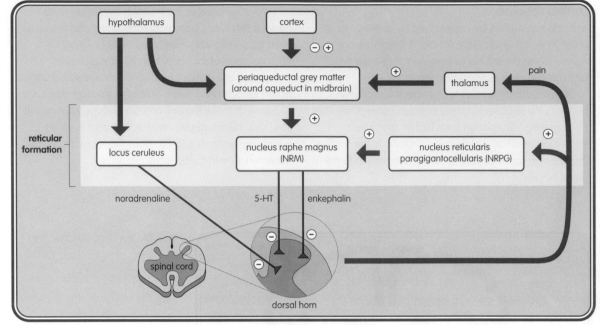

Fig. 3.14 Central regulation of pain.

There are three classes of endogenous opioid peptides that contain the amino-acid sequence of either leucine–enkephalin (Tyr-Gly-Gly-Phe-Leu) or methionine–enkephalin (Tyr-Gly-Gly-Phe-Met). Fig. 3.15 shows the different sizes of opioid peptide, their parent peptide sequences and their distribution.

There are three major classes of opioid receptor:

- μ
- δ
- κ

Morphine is a potent μ agonist and naloxone an antagonist. Endogenous enkephalins are active at both μ and δ receptors. Both receptor types are found in the periaqueductal grey matter and in laminae I and II of the dorsal horn.

Note that each of these receptors is found throughout the central nervous system, suggesting that they are involved in processes other than pain perception.

Analgesia

Analgesia is relief from the psychological state of pain. The main analgesics in clinical use are:

- Opioid analgesics acting on the endogenous system of pain control.
- Non-steroidal anti-inflammatory drugs, which reduce the production of inflammatory mediators

that sensitize nociceptors to bradykinin and 5-HT.
- Local anaesthetics, which block action potential conduction along axons.
- Miscellaneous drugs, e.g. sumatriptan (5-HT$_{1D}$ agonist) in migraine, carbamazepine (antiepileptic) in trigeminal neuralgia, tricyclic antidepressants (amitryptyline) in chronic pain.

Opioids

Opioid drugs bind to the receptors of the endogenous opioid transmitters. There are two classes of opioids:

- Opiates, which are morphine analogues with structures like morphine and usually synthesized from it. Fig. 3.16 shows the structure of morphine with two coplanar rings at a right angle to another two coplanar rings.
- Synthetic derivatives structurally unrelated to morphine.

In the antinociceptive system, opioids will block pain information from being transmitted up the spinothalamic tract (antinociceptive action) but they also act in the brain to reduce the unpleasantness of the pain state (analgesic action).

The main effect of opioids is on the μ receptor, causing:

- Analgesia and antinociception.

Opioid peptides			
Parent peptide	**Opioid peptide**	**Amino acid sequence**	**Location**
proenkephalin	enkephalins	Leu^5, Met^5, and longer sequences	spinal cord, brainstem
prodynorphin	dynorphins	all contain Leu^5 within longer sequences	spinal cord, brainstem
pro-opiomelanocortin	β endorphin	Met^5 in 31 amino acid sequence	hypothalamus

Fig. 3.15 Opioid peptides.

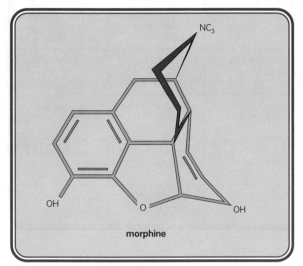

Fig. 3.16 Structure of morphine.

- Euphoria (sense of wellbeing)—depending on circumstances of administration.
- Respiratory depression—reducing sensitivity of brainstem to P_aCO_2.
- Miosis—pupillary constriction caused by stimulation of parasympathetic component of cranial nerve III.
- Emesis—stimulation of chemoreceptor trigger zone in the brainstem which sends signals to the vomiting centre.
- Constipation—increased tone and reduced motility of gastrointestinal tract.

The opiate class of opioids (morphine, diamorphine, codeine) also cause histamine release from mast cells and are cough suppressants, but these effects are not mediated by opioid receptors.

There are problems with repeated administration of opioids:
- Tolerance—a gradual reduction in effect over repeated administration of the same amount of drug. Tolerance is high to analgesia and emesis, low to miosis and constipation.
- Dependence—this can be physical (where a withdrawal syndrome of physical symptoms and signs like flu occurs when the drug is not administered) or psychological (where compulsive drug-seeking behaviour develops).

The main danger of opioid abuse is from overdose, which presents with:
- Coma, respiratory depression (reduced ventilation as decreased sensitivity to P_aCO_2) and pin-point pupils (there is no tolerance to pupillary constriction even in the hardened addict).
- Treatment is with intravenous μ-antagonists, which reverse the effects of opioids such as naloxone (rapidly acting and short duration of action) or naltrexone (longer to act but longer duration of action). Note that antagonists may stimulate an acute withdrawal state and supportive therapy alone (e.g. ventilation) may be appropriate.

The main opioids are shown in Fig. 3.17 with their different pharmacological properties and clinical uses.

Non-steroidal anti-inflammatory drugs
Non-steroidal anti-inflammatory drugs (NSAIDs) relieve pain by reducing the sensitization of nociceptors that occurs in inflammation. They inhibit cyclooxygenase (which metabolizes arachidonic acid to prostaglandins) and leukotrienes (which have roles in continuing the process of inflammation). NSAIDs are also anti-inflammatory and antipyretic.

The prostaglandins, PGE$_1$ and PGE$_2$, lower the threshold of polymodal nociceptors to stimulation by the inflammatory mediators bradykinin and 5-HT.

Side effects of these drugs can result from interference with the physiological role of

Opioid drugs					
μ Agonist	Bioavailability and administraion	Metabolism	Potency and length of action	Clinical use	Notes
morphine	Poor orally, involved in enterohepatic recirculation. Intravenous administration gives reliable dosing	active metabolite morphine-6-glucuronide	$t_{1/2}$ 3 h	acute and chronic pain	cannot be given in labour as fetal liver cannot conjugate
diamorphine (heroin)	More lipid soluble. Given orally or by intramuscular, intravenous or subcutaneous injection	partly to morphine	very potent, rapid onset, $t_{1/2}$ 2 hrs	acute and chronic pain	
codeine	High oral bioavailability	to other opioids including morphine	one-sixth potency of morphine	mild pain, headache, dental pain	potent antitussive, low side effect profile
pethidine	High lipid solubility. Given orally and by intramuscular injection	metabolite norpethidine interacts with MAOIs	one-tenth potency of morphine	acute pain, labour	does not cause miosis
fentanyl	High lipid solubility. Given intravenously, epidurally, transdermally		very potent, short acting	intra-operative pain	intra-operative analgesia
buprenorphine	Increased first-pass metabolism. Given sublingually, intra-thecally		$t_{1/2}$ 12 h, slow onset	acute and chronic pain	partial agonist and difficult to reverse effects in overdose
methadone	Given orally or by injection		$t_{1/2}$ >24 h, very slow onset	maintenance of drug addicts	does not produce euphoria

Fig. 3.17 Opioid drugs. (MAOI, monoamine oxiidase inhibitors.)

prostaglandins in the regulation of blood flow. The production of prostaglandins in these normal circumstances is by a subtype of cyclooxygenase, cyclooxygenase-1. The other type, cyclooxygenase-2, is inducible and metabolizes arachidonic acid in inflammatory cells. Interfering with prostaglandin-mediated blood flow, in the gastric mucosa for example, reduces HCO_3^- production and gastric acid can then attack the mucosal surface causing ulceration.

Fig. 3.18 shows the main NSAIDs in clinical use with their effects and side effects, and Fig. 3.19 shows the site of action of NSAIDs.

Local anaesthetic agents

Local anaesthetic agents block the ability of axons to conduct action potentials by blocking Na^+ channels in the axonal membrane. They are weak bases that can exist, depending on their *pK*, in either a hydrophilic state, when bound to H^+, or in hydrophobic state without H^+.

- In the hydrophobic state they can pass through the lipid membrane into the axon or straight into the channel through its walls which lie in the membrane, whether the channel is closed or open.
- In the hydrophilic state they can enter only from the inside of the axon through the open mouth of the channel and therefore need to wait until the channel opens. The hydrophilic route of the drug to plug the channel leads to 'use-dependent' block—the block of channels increases as more channels open.

Fig. 3.20 shows both hydrophilic (XH^+) and hydrophobic (X) blocking of a Na^+ channel.

At low concentrations of local anaesthetic agents, only small-diameter myelinated and unmyelinated fibres are affected. This means that administration of local anaesthetic agents can be used to produce a differential nerve block affecting only Aδ and C fibres. This reduces pain and temperature transmission, leaving proprioception, fine touch, and motor functions intact.

Non-steroidal anti-inflammatory drugs	
Drug	**Uses and side effects of NSAIDs**
aspirin	drug of choice for mild pain; causes gastrointestinal upset, haemorrhage, salicylism (tinnitus, dizziness, nausea), Reye's syndrome in children (postviral encephalopathy and liver disorder)
paracetamol	no great analgesic effect in inflammatory conditions but efficacious for headache; liver failure in overdose
ibuprofen	inflammatory joint disease, dental pain; much milder side effect profile
mefenamic acid	moderately effective; causes gastrointestinal tract upset and diarrhoea

Fig. 3.18 Uses and side effects of non-steroidal anti-inflammatory drugs (NSAIDs).

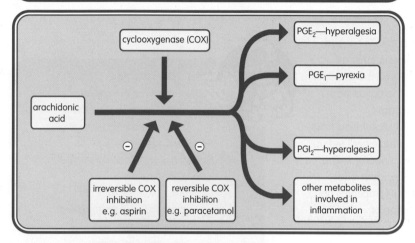

Fig. 3.19 Site of action of NSAIDs. (COX, cyclooxygenase.)

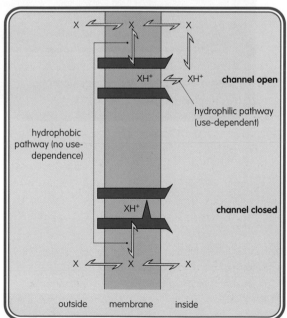

Fig. 3.20 Mechanism of action of local anaesthetics. Local anaesthetic agents (X) can interact with channels. This is either by the hydrophilic pathway through the open channel by a charged species (XH^+) or directly from the membrane by the uncharged species (X) by the hydrophobic pathway.

To increase the effect of a given amount of local anaesthetic agent, a vasoconstrictor (e.g. adrenaline) can be given with the local anaesthetic to reduce the rate at which the local anaesthetic is washed out of the tissue being anaesthetized. This is not advisable when the tissue being anaesthetized relies on end arteries for supply (e.g. digital arteries in fingers and toes) because ischaemic necrosis will result.

The common local anaesthetic agents in use are shown in Fig. 3.21

Chronic pain

Chronic pain is pain that continues when the causative stimulus is no longer present. Characteristic features are:

- Hyperalgesia—more pain is felt for a given amount of noxious stimulation.
- Allodynia—pain caused by innocuous stimuli.
- Spontaneous pain spasms—pain felt in the absence of any stimulation.

The chronic pain state is caused by a hyperactive acute pain pathway.

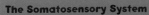

Local anaesthetic agents		
Drug	Use	Side effects
lignocaine	nerve-block anaesthesia, e.g. dentistry; spinal anaesthesia—injection into subarachnoid space for surgery to lower trunk and legs	spinal procedure affects many nerve roots—hypotension and bradycardia caused by sympathetic block, urinary retention caused by block of pelvic autonomic fibres
bupivacaine	epidural anaesthesia to block spinal roots for pain of labour	less than for spinal, as injection into epidural space minimizes diffusion to other nerve roots

Fig. 3.21 Local anaesthetic agents.

Increased responsiveness of nociceptors is caused by sensitization by inflammatory mediators such as bradykinin, prostaglandins, and nerve growth factor.

Increased excitability of neurons in the dorsal horn and thalamus is due to increases in synaptic transmission that occur after prolonged stimulation. This means that high nociceptor firing frequencies will set up a state of hyperexcitability in dorsal horn neurons. The process that facilitates this increase in synaptic effect involves the NMDA (N-methyl-D-aspartate) receptor and NMDA antagonists can block the initiation of hyperexcitability.

Neurological disease can affect the pain pathway and produce neuropathic pain, a form of chronic pain caused by damaged sensory neurons. Often, α-adrenergic receptors are expressed on the neurons and as a result sympathetic activity can cause severe pain.

Psychological aspects of pain

There are many social and psychological influences on pain perception and pain behaviour. Chronic pain that is resistant to any drug therapy may be treated by psychological methods.

- Discuss the pain/nociception distinction. List the characteristics of nociceptors.
- Summarize the processing of nociceptive signals.
- Explain the efficacy of opioid drugs as analgesics.
- Describe the use, side effects, and treatment of overdose of opioid drugs.
- Describe the use and side effects of NSAIDs and local anaesthetics.
- Discuss the mechanisms of chronic pain.

4. Motor Control

MOVEMENT CONTROL

Types of movement

There are three basic types of movement.

- Reflex responses (e.g. the gag reflex)—simple stereotyped involuntary responses graded to the eliciting stimulus.
- Rhythmic motor patterns (e.g. walking)—sequences of stereotyped repetitive responses that require voluntary control to start and stop.
- Voluntary movements—these are goal directed, usually learnt, and improve with practice.

The importance of sensation

Sensory information can be used in a feedback or feed-forward control system.

- In feedback control, the nervous system generates a desired output and sensory information is used to obtain an error signal, which is the desired position minus the current position. In patients with large-fibre sensory neuropathy, unless they can see their limbs they do not know where they are in space.
- In feed-forward control, sensory information is used to derive advance information and direct the movement towards a predicted position (e.g. catching objects).

Motor programmes and voluntary movement

Definitions

A 'motor programme' is a set of commands that, when sent to a group of muscles, will execute a movement. The same motor programme can be scaled and timed differently and sent to different muscle groups—consider that we can write our signature with our hands or our feet. A motor programme is an abstract concept that helps us to understand how the motor system executes movement.

A 'motor strategy' is a set of motor programmes that have been selected and sequenced to achieve a recognized goal.

Development of motor programmes

Motor programmes are time-saving for the motor system because they enable fast accurate movement. They need to be learned because proprioceptive feedback is not used in their execution, although motor output is always checked using feedback.

The following stages in the process of learning motor programmes show how proprioceptive feedback is used to adjust the motor output until the precise motor commands are developed.

- As a motor task is learned, the pattern of muscle activity changes. Initially, discontinuous movement occurs where agonist muscles only move the limb nearer and nearer towards a target, judging the end-point with feedback.
- Then faster continuous movement develops, with a single agonist burst stopped by an antagonist, then smaller adjustments guided by feedback made with agonist muscles.
- Eventually, the movement becomes ballistic, with a single agonist burst to move the limb towards the target and a single antagonist burst to stop the limb moving so that it comes to rest at the target.

Fig. 4.1 shows the electromyogram (EMG) activity for each stage of motor learning.

Hierarchy of movement control

There are three levels of motor control arranged hierarchically and in parallel. The lowest level is at the spinal cord. The interneurons in the cord play a major role in sequential operations of muscles which can produce complex movements under sensory control.

The intermediate level is at the brainstem containing medial, lateral, and aminergic systems. These project to and regulate segmental networks of the spinal cord and are responsible for the integration of visual, vestibular, and somatosensory inputs in the control of posture. Also, some brainstem nuclei control eye and head movements.

The highest level is in the control of voluntary movement.

- Processes that generate the desire to move in response to recognized demands can be localized to the frontal lobes and limbic system.

- Processes generating strategies to achieve motor aims, by selecting motor programmes, can be localized to the complex of the premotor and supplementary motor areas. Each area projects onto the primary motor cortex and spinal motor neurons via the corticospinal tract and indirectly via the brainstem, and is also arranged somatotopically both for input and output. The basal ganglia also have a role in motor planning in the scaling and initiation of motor programmes.

- Processes that guide movement are carried out by the primary motor cortex and descending motor tracts. The pyramidal tract governs highly skilled movement involving few muscles. The cerebellum improves the accuracy of movements by comparing descending motor commands with information about resulting motor activity.

- The process of execution of movement is carried out by spinal cells that innervate skeletal muscle.

- **How is proprioceptive information used in the development of motor programmes.**
- **Discuss the hierarchical control of voluntary movement. How can it be localized?**
- **Discuss the importance of proprioceptive feedback in the control of movement and in performing highly skilled movements.**

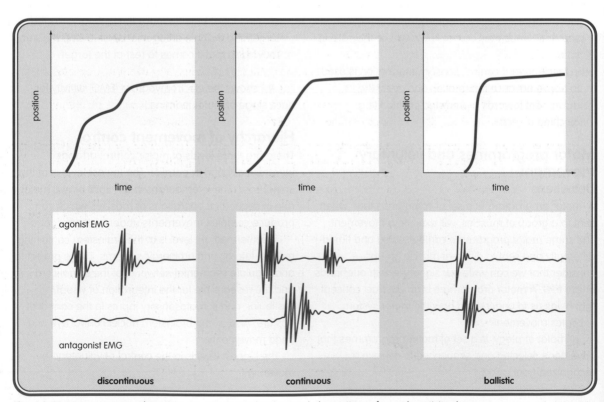

Fig. 4.1 Motor programme learning. As a motor task is learned, the pattern of muscle activity changes.

MOTOR UNITS AND RECRUITMENT OF MUSCLE FIBRES

Motor units

A motor unit consists of a motor neuron and all the muscle fibres that it innervates. One motor neuron may innervate many fibres but a single fibre receives input from only one motor neuron (Fig. 4.2).

The innervation ratio of a motor unit is the number of fibres that its motor neuron innervates. A high innervation ratio means that one motor neuron controls many fibres—such a motor unit produces coarse strong movements (e.g. the motor units in gastrocnemius have a ratio of 2000:1). A low innervation ratio means that only a few fibres are controlled by a motor neuron—such a motor unit produces fine well-controlled movement (e.g. the motor units in the extraocular muscles have a ratio of 10:1).

Motor units differ in their properties owing to variation in types of motor neuron and variation in types of fibre innervated.

Recruitment

Recruitment describes the order in which types of motor units are activated when making any movement, whether it is reflex or voluntary. Slow units are activated first, then fast fatigue-resistant units, and then fast-fatiguable units.

This allows the motor system to grade simply the amount of force used in a movement. A small amount of excitatory input to a pool of different types of motor neurons in the anterior horn will only produce firing of the slow-unit motor neurons. Greater amounts of stimulation are required to activate the faster and more powerful units.

The order of activation in recruitment may be explained by motor neuron size. Slow-unit motor neurons have smaller cell bodies and therefore a lower surface area. A lower surface area increases the resistance of the neuron to input currents. With a high resistance, a greater potential is generated for a given amount of input current. This means that a small amount of excitatory input may activate small motor neurons but not be great enough to depolarize larger motor neurons.

Tetany

Tetanic contraction occurs when successive muscle contractions are so rapid that they fuse together resulting in a sustained maximally forceful contraction. This phenomenon is seen *in vitro*.

Tetany occurs where hypocalcaemia or alkalosis reduce the threshold for action potential generation and neurons fire spontaneously, producing a characteristic spasm of the hands with the fingers and thumbs adducted and hand flexed at the metacarpophalangeal joints.

Responses of motor units in damage and disease

The different types of motor units are present in equal amounts and spread out evenly in most muscles, as seen by staining techniques that pick up enzyme quantities (e.g. myosin ATPase).

Properties of motor neurons and function, histology, and biochemistry of muscle fibres			
Motor unit	Properties of motor neuron	Functional properties of muscle fibres	Histology and biochemistry of muscle fibres
fast fatiguable	progressive drop in firing rate with steady-state depolarization; large cell body, large-diameter axon with high conduction velocity	fast contraction and relaxation times, high force during tetanus, fatigue after repeated stimulation	few mitochondria, high levels of glycolytic enzymes (phosphorylase), high levels of myosin ATPase
slow fatigue-resistant	constant low-frequency firing rate with steady-state depolarization; smaller cell body, smaller diameter axon with slower conduction velocity	longer contraction and relaxation times, lower force (10% of fast fatiguable), very resistant to fatigue	many mitochondria, high levels of oxidative enzymes (succinic dehydrogenase), high levels of myoglobin
fast fatigue-resistant	intermediate firing rate response to steady-state depolarization; intermediate cell body size, axon diameter and conduction speed	slightly slower than fast fatiguable contraction and relaxation times, twice force of slow units, very resistant to fatigue	many mitochondria, high levels of glycolytic and oxidative enzymes, high levels of myosin ATPase

Fig. 4.2 Properties of motoneurons and function, histology, and biochemistry of muscle fibres.

49

Clinical features and effects on motor units of diseases of the motor neuron cell body, peripheral axon, and muscle fibre				
Part of motor unit affected	Typical clinical features	Example	Effect on muscle fibres	EMG changes
motor neuron cell body	weakness, atrophy affecting distal muscles more than proximal, fasciculation [lower motor neuron lesion signs although hyperreflexia is seen in amyotrophic lateral sclerosis (ALS)]	amyotrophic lateral sclerosis	atrophy and disappearance of groups of muscle fibres, with other fibres innervated by new collaterals from remaining motor neurons; this produces 'fibre clumping' where areas of muscle contain fibres of only one type (fibre type is determined by motor neuron type—response to disease results in collaterals of one motor neuron innervating many nearby fibres)	spontaneous activity at rest (fibrillation), discrete pattern of potentials during voluntary contraction as fewer motor units active, potentials are larger as motor units innervate more fibres than usual; no change in axon conduction velocity
motor neuron axon	chronically—weakness, atrophy distally, loss of tendon reflexes, sensory symptoms (loss, paraesthesia) as all types of peripheral nerve are affected	Guillain–Barré syndrome		fibrillation, discrete large potentials; demyelinating neuropathies (Guillain–Barré syndrome) result in reduced axon conduction velocity
muscle fibre	weakness initially affecting walking and lifting, proximal larger muscles involved more than distal ones	Duchenne's muscular dystrophy	no change in spread of type of motor unit; dead fibres and regenerating fibres are present; inflammatory cells and fat sometimes present	no spontaneous activity at rest, shorter smaller potentials as there are fewer remaining fibres in each motor unit; the overall pattern is still smooth as there is no reduction in the number of motor units firing

Fig. 4.3 Clinical features and effects on motor units of diseases of the motor neuron cell body, peripheral axon, and muscle fibre.

Diseases affecting the different parts of the motor unit disrupt the normal function of motor units, as shown by changes in the pattern of motor unit arrangement, the size of muscle fibres, and electrical recordings from muscle when active and at rest (electromyogram).

The clinical features and effects on motor units of diseases of the motor neuron cell body, peripheral axon, and muscle fibre are shown in Fig. 4.3

- ○ **What is a motor unit?**
- ○ **Explain the variation in function of motor units in terms of innervation ratios and enzyme content.**
- ○ **Explain the function of recruitment.**
- ○ **Describe the histological, biochemical, and electromyographic changes that occur in diseases of the motor unit. Relate these to the clinical findings.**

REFLEX ACTION AND MUSCLE TONE

Clinical relevance

Neurological examination of patients begins with testing stretch reflexes. Tapping the patella tendon and observing the results tells you whether the spinal cord segments L2 and L3 are intact, excluding peripheral nerve damage, and can also indicate if the spinal motor neurons are receiving an abnormal drive.

Passive movement of a limb tells the examiner about the tone of the muscles in the limb.

Definitions

'Reflex action' is an automatic motor response (simple or highly coordinated) that is elicited by a stimulus. The stretch reflex is simple because the stretch detector (the muscle spindle) makes a monosynaptic connection with the output spinal motor neuron. Other reflexes have neurons between the sensory input and the motor output (interneurons) and can produce more complex responses.

'Muscle tone' is the resting tension in muscle. It is produced by tonic firing of spinal motor neurons and their firing frequency is set by various inputs from stretch receptors and from higher centres through corticospinal, vestibulospinal, cerebellospinal, and rubrospinal tracts.

In parkinsonism there is 'rigidity' where all muscles have increased tone but there is no change in the strength of the reflexes. Thus there is no alteration in the reflex circuit but there is an alteration in the direct corticospinal input.

After cell death in the motor cortex in a 'stroke' caused by haemorrhage or ischaemia, there is 'spasticity' on the contralateral side, where tone is increased more in limb flexors than extensors and stretch reflexes elicit stronger responses. In this case a reduced cortical input to the reflex circuit frees it from inhibition and its activity is increased, both at rest and when appropriately stimulated.

Proprioceptors and reflexes
Muscle spindles

Spindles consist of muscle fibres enclosed in a connective tissue capsule (the fibres are termed 'intrafusal' muscle fibres; all the normal fibres lying outside the spindles are termed 'extrafusal'). Only the ends of these fibres can contract.

Sensory endings from dorsal root ganglion cells enter the capsule and innervate the non-contractile middle part of these fibres. Different types of fibres are named according to the appearance of their nuclei, either lying in a chain along the fibre or clumped as a bag of nuclei in the middle as shown in Fig. 4.4.

The function of the spindle is to provide information about muscle length and velocity of change in length. Two types of sensory ending from the spindle encode this information and their properties are compared in Fig. 4.5.

The contractile parts of the intrafusal fibres are innervated by γ-motor neurons which serve to alter the sensitivity of the fibres to stretch and to velocity. Dynamic γ-motor neurons innervate dynamic bag fibres and static γ-motor neurons innervate static bag and chain fibres.

Spindles and α-motor neuron firing

Increasing the activity of γ-motor neurons contracts the ends of the intrafusal fibres thereby stretching the middle of the fibres. The middle is innervated by stretch-receptor afferent nerves which are connected to α-motor neurons. Therefore, α-motor neurons can be made to discharge by activation of γ-motor neurons through the reflex loop.

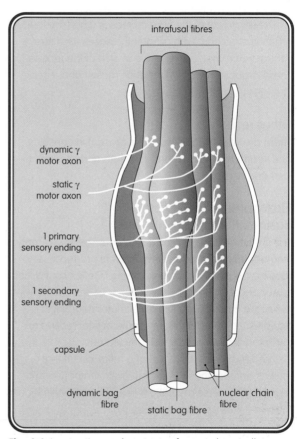

Fig. 4.4 Innervation and contents of a muscle spindle.

Fig. 4.5 Properties of the two types of sensory ending from the muscle spindle.

Properties of the two types of sensory ending from the muscle spindle			
Type	**Contact**	**Response to linear stretch**	**Encoding**
Ia (primary) ending	dynamic bag, static bag, nuclear chain	dynamic　　　　static action potentials	velocity of change of length, static length
II (secondary) ending	static bag, nuclear chain	dynamic　　　　static time ⟶	static length

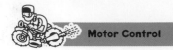

Also, α-motor neurons and γ-motor neurons are often activated together, so that the muscle spindle is very sensitive when the muscle is in use, and this provides very accurate feedback for error detection in voluntary movement.

Golgi tendon organs

Golgi tendon organs are composed of a network of collagen fibres inside a connective tissue capsule with a sensory axon winding around the collagen.

The firing rate of the fibre increases when the tendon organ is stretched, with greater increases for active contraction rather than passive stretch of the muscle. These organs provide information mainly about active changes in tension in the muscle.

Other receptors

There are various joint receptors present in capsules and ligaments that respond to length and changes in joint angle.

Examples of reflexes
Basic pattern

The stretch reflex is elicited when a muscle is suddenly lengthened and a reflex contraction is produced (e.g. tapping the patellar tendon causing a reflex contraction of quadriceps). Homonymous motor neurons (supplying the same muscle) and synergist motor neurons (supplying a muscle with the same action) receive an excitatory input from the spindle afferent.

Tendon organs form part of a reflex circuit that inhibits homonymous and synergistic motor neurons, termed the inverse myotatic reflex. The pathways for these reflexes are shown in Fig. 4.6

Blink reflex

The blink reflex protects the cornea from foreign bodies (Fig. 4.7). All other reflexes listed below are more complex, involving the coordination of a number of muscle groups.

Gag reflex (Fig. 4.8)

This reflex protects the alimentary tract and upper airway from foreign bodies.

Flexion withdrawal reflex

The flexion withdrawal reflex is a more complicated motor act that protects limbs against noxious stimuli detected by cutaneous structures. The flexors of the affected limb contract and the extensors are relaxed. This withdraws the limb away from the noxious stimulus.

At the same time, a crossed extensor reflex is elicited in the contralateral limb where the extensors are contracted and the flexors relaxed. This provides postural support during the withdrawal of the stimulated limb.

Fig. 4.9 shows the polysynaptic pathways in the spinal cord with extensor and flexor action of stimulated and nonstimulated limbs.

Plantar reflex

The plantar reflex is elicited when the plantar surface of the foot is stroked from heel to toe, causing reflex plantar flexion of the toes in normal individuals. However, in infants (whose corticospinal tract is not yet fully myelinated) and in patients with damage to the motor cortex or corticospinal tract, dorsiflexion of the toes is elicited.

- What is a reflex?
- Describe how the different afferent nerves from muscle spindles give information about length change, velocity, and position.
- Describe how the sensitivity of the spindles can be altered.
- Describe the influences on muscle tone.
- Compare the function of tendon organs and muscle spindles with reference to their involvement in spinal reflexes.
- Describe the anatomical basis of reflexes involving the cord (flexion withdrawal) and the brainstem (blink and gag).

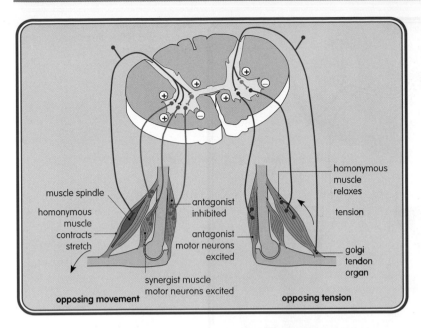

Fig. 4.6 Muscle spindle and Golgi tendon organ reflexes—opposite effects.

muscle spindle

homonymous muscle contracts stretch

antagonist inhibited

antagonist motor neurons excited

synergist muscle motor neurons excited

opposing movement

homonymous muscle relaxes

tension

golgi tendon organ

opposing tension

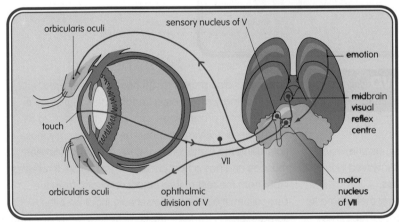

Fig. 4.7 Corneal (blink) reflex. This blink reflex protects the cornea from foreign bodies.

orbicularis oculi

sensory nucleus of V

emotion

midbrain visual reflex centre

touch

motor nucleus of VII

orbicularis oculi

ophthalmic division of V

VII

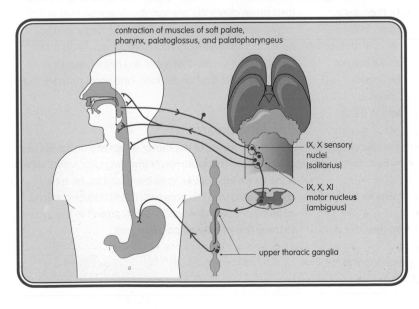

Fig. 4.8 Gag reflex showing a combination of skeletal muscle and smooth muscle action.

contraction of muscles of soft palate, pharynx, palatoglossus, and palatopharyngeus

IX, X sensory nuclei (solitarius)

IX, X, XI motor nucleus (ambiguus)

upper thoracic ganglia

53

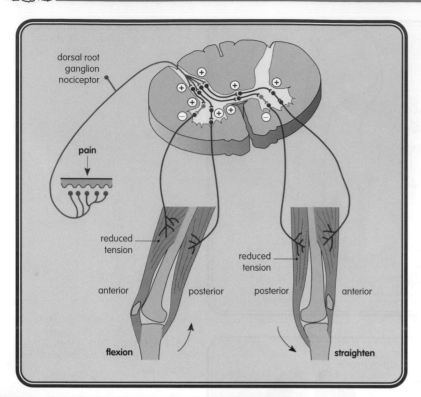

Fig. 4.9 Circuitry of the flexion withdrawal reflex, for muscles acting at the knee.

dorsal root
ganglion
nociceptor

pain

reduced
tension

reduced
tension

anterior

posterior

posterior

anterior

flexion

straighten

THE MOTOR CORTEX AND PYRAMIDAL TRACTS

The motor cortex

The motor cortex lying in the frontal lobe, as shown in Fig. 4.10, is the area of the cortex that is involved in the planning and output of motor commands.

The premotor area and supplementary motor area lie next to the primary motor area in the frontal lobe. They plan movements, as suggested by positron emission tomography scanning where increased metabolism is seen in the premotor area and supplementary motor area when subjects are asked to think about but not execute a movement. These areas are arranged according to a body plan, a motor homunculus:

- The supplementary motor area projects to distal muscles.
- The premotor area projects through the reticulospinal tract to proximal muscles.

Both areas receive input from motor regions that process different aspects of movement:

- The premotor area receives input from the cerebellum via the thalamus.
- The supplementary motor area receives input from the basal ganglia through the thalamus.

Both areas also project to the primary motor area.

The primary motor area performs the final stage in cortical motor processing—execution. It projects to all contralateral body motor neurons but principally those controlling the digits, toes, and facial and vocalization muscles and has a homuncular organization. It receives input from the rest of the motor cortex and from the cerebellum. It also receives sensory input from the somatosensory cortex—the cortical area for muscle and joint sense abuts the primary motor cortex.

Movements are represented in the motor cortex homunculi and although the homunculus is an artistic abstraction it shows that there is a higher repertoire of movements for the hands, face, and vocal muscles than for the trunk.

Cellular organization

The cellular layers of the motor cortex are unlike the rest of the cortex. The fourth layer (the 'granular' layer), which is the major input layer, is missing and so the motor cortex is said to be 'agranular'. The fifth layer contains large output cells (Betz cells) which project to the cord, forming 12% of the corticospinal tract.

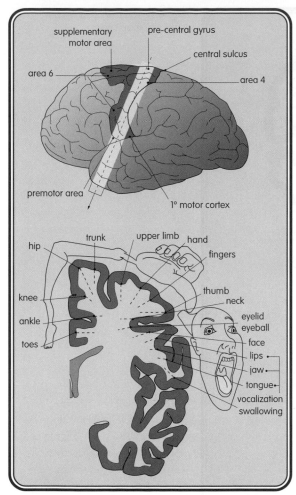

Fig. 4.10 Location and homuncular organization of the motor cortex.

Further clues to functional organization
In epilepsy, disordered neuronal firing during a fit can affect the motor cortex. This produces a wave of muscle activity, termed a 'jacksonian march', that moves over the body as the disruption of function spreads over the motor cortex. This partly led to theories of homuncular organization of the motor cortex.

The pyramidal tract (corticospinal tract)

Fig. 4.11 shows the cortical origins of the tract and the termination pattern of the lateral tract to lateral limb muscle motor neuron pools and the anterior tract to anterior axial muscle motor neuron pools.

The fibres that influence motor neurons innervating muscles in the head (e.g. extraocular muscles, tongue muscles, and facial muscles) run in the corticobulbar tracts to the appropriate cranial nerve nuclei. The somatotopic arrangement of the descending motor fibres from the cortex includes the head in the cerebral peduncles, but not at the level of decussation in the medulla.

The motor fibres carry signals for highly skilled voluntary movements. To achieve this:
- The tract needs to be highly somatotopic.
- The fibres must have few collaterals so that excitation from one fibre is communicated to the minimum number of spinal motor neurons (this allows a great deal of control over the execution of movement).

As well as motor axons, there are fibres that regulate spinal reflexes in the tract and feedback to the dorsal horn sensory circuits from the sensory cortex.

Upper and lower motor neuron lesions

Damage to the motor cortex gives absence of volitional movement but experimental evidence from cutting just the pyramidal tract in the medulla of monkeys gives very little motor deficit.

In humans, damage to the motor cortex after a cerebrovascular accident (ischaemic or haemorrhagic) leads to a set of symptoms and signs affecting some of the contralateral muscles in the limbs and face. Because upper (i.e. cortical) motor neurons are involved, the effect is termed an 'upper motor neuron lesion', although other cells are involved too.

Voluntary paresis (weakness) is caused by loss of corticospinal input. Spasticity or abnormal distribution in muscle tone affects flexors more than extensors, but this may be caused by disruption of extrapyramidal systems.

The following signs are caused by disruption of the descending influence on reflex circuits:
- Stronger deep reflexes (e.g. knee jerk).
- Loss of superficial reflexes (e.g. abdominal, cremasteric).

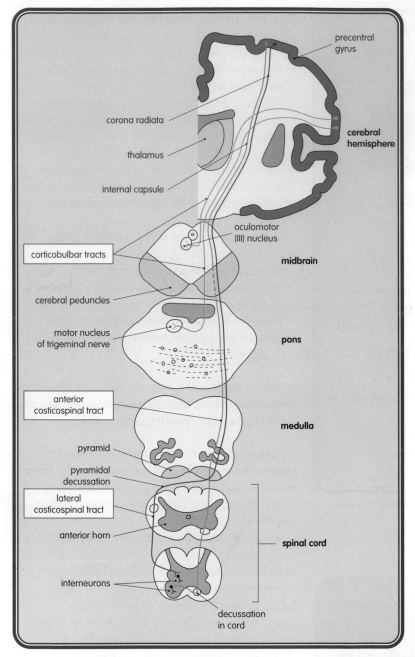

Fig. 4.11 The corticospinal and corticobulbar tracts.

precentral gyrus

corona radiata

thalamus

internal capsule

cerebral hemisphere

oculomotor (III) nucleus

corticobulbar tracts

midbrain

cerebral peduncles

motor nucleus of trigeminal nerve

pons

anterior costicospinal tract

medulla

pyramid

pyramidal decussation

lateral costicospinal tract

anterior horn

spinal cord

interneurons

decussation in cord

• Positive Babinski's sign—extensor plantar response to stroking the lateral part of the sole from heel to toe.

The effects of an upper motor neuron lesion are typically seen on one side of the body contralateral to the lesion. If there is localized damage to the motor cortex or pyramidal tract, all the input to an area will be affected due to homuncular and somatotopic organization.

Fig. 4.12 compares the effect of disruption in the anterior and middle cerebral arteries.

Damage to the spinal motor neurons either in the cord or along their pathway to the site of innervation of the muscle produces a different set of symptoms and signs, referred to as a lower motor neuron lesion:
• Weakness caused by loss of nervous innervation.
• Atrophy as a result of disuse.
• Fasciculation (squirming movements of the muscle) caused by increased sensitivity at receptor level to any acetylcholine that is released from intact terminals.
• Absent reflexes caused by loss of reflex output.

A comparison of the effects of disruption in the anterior and middle cerebral arteries			
Artery	Region supplied	Part of homunculus supplied	Effect of haemorrhage
anterior cerebral	medial part of primary motor cortex	lower limb	upper motor neuron (UMN) lesion of lower limb
middle cerebral	lateral part of primary motor cortex, internal capsule	head and upper limb	cortex: UMN lesion of upper limb and face internal capsule: damage to motor and sensory fibres

Fig. 4.12 A comparison of the effects of disruption in the anterior and middle cerebral arteries.

- Where are the motor cortex and its subdivisions?
- State the functions of the motor cortex subdivisions in terms of planning and execution.
- Describe the homuncular organization of the motor cortex.
- Describe the path of the pyramidal tract and its function in relation to the cells of origin in the tract and their termination in the cord.
- Relate the signs of an upper motor neuron lesion to pyramidal tract function and compare these with the signs of a lower motor neuron lesion.

BASAL GANGLIA AND THALAMUS

Overview

The basal ganglia consist of five nuclei with extensive connections and they are involved in motor control and cognition. They are functionally inserted in a processing loop with the cortex and thalamus. Basal ganglia function is further understood by relating the signs of Parkinson's and Huntington's disease to the affected parts of the basal ganglia.

Anatomy

Fig. A1.3 (Appendix 1) shows the relationship between the putamen, caudate nucleus, and all the elements of the basal ganglia.

Fig. 4.13 shows the thalamus as a rugby ball-shaped collection of cell groups with thalami on either side connected (by the interthalamic connexus).

The thalamus is organized around a Y-shaped collection of white matter called the 'internal medullary lamina'. This splits the thalamus into three

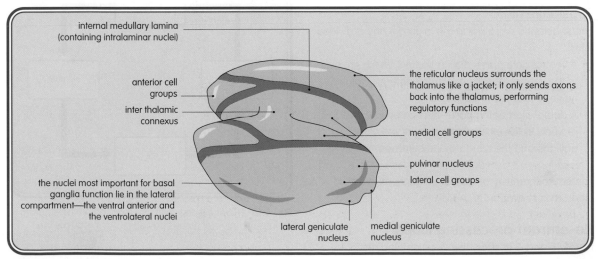

Fig. 4.13 The thalamus.

sections—the anterior, lateral, and medial sections. Each section is composed of numerous cell groups with particular inputs and functions, and there are also cell groups inside the medullary lamina (the intralaminar nuclei).

Connections and circuits of the basal ganglia and thalamus

Caudate and putamen

The caudate and putamen contain identical cell types and together they form the neostriatum. They receive information from motor, sensory, association, and limbic areas.

The corticostriate projection is topographically and functionally organized so that the putamen is concerned with motor control and the caudate with eye movements and cognition. They project to the globus pallidus and subthalamic nucleus. The putamen also sends a projection to the pars reticulata of the substantia nigra.

Globus pallidus

The globus pallidus is divided into internal (GP$_i$) and external (GP$_e$) segments lying lateral to the internal capsule and medial to the putamen. The internal segment is the major output nucleus projecting to the ventral lateral and ventral anterior nuclei of the thalamus.

Subthalamic nucleus

The subthalamic nucleus lies below the thalamus at its junction with the midbrain and receives a projection from and projects back to the external segment of the globus pallidus.

Substantia nigra

The substantia nigra lies in the midbrain and is divided into:

- A ventral pale part—pars reticulata, which projects to the ventral lateral and ventral anterior thalamic nuclei, the superior colliculus.
- A dorsal pigmented part—pars compacta, which projects to the external segment of the globus pallidus and the caudate and putamen.

The neurochemistry of cellular interactions in the striatum is shown in Fig. 4.14.

Re-entrant processing loops

Figs 4.15 and 4.16 show the direct and indirect processing loops that run through the basal ganglia. If you work through each loop looking at the patterns of excitation and inhibition, the direct loop excites the cortex and the indirect loop inhibits.

Functions of the basal ganglia

The basal ganglia select the motor programmes that are appropriate for a particular task that involves cognitive processing and motor processing. They affect the processing of stimuli for movement and the initiation of movement.

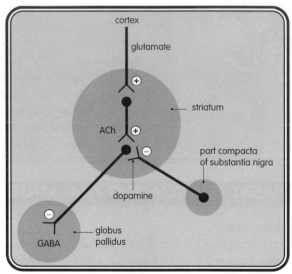

Fig. 4.14 Influences on striatal output—neurochemical connections. (ACh, acetylcholine; GABA, γ-aminobutyric acid.)

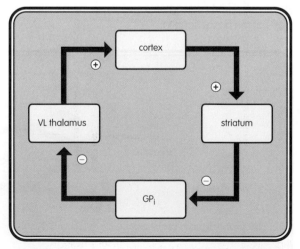

Fig. 4.15 The direct corticostriatal loop. When the striatum inhibits the internal globus pallidus (GP$_i$), it reduces the ability of the GP$_i$ to inhibit the thalamus. This frees the thalamus to excite the cortex (supplementary motor area). (VL, ventrolateral.)

They scale the output of the motor programme so that appropriate movements are made. This is particularly important in motor programmes with fine movement (e.g. handwriting) and also where similar repetitive movements are needed (e.g. in locomotion).

Disorders involving basal ganglia function and their treatment
Parkinsonism
The signs resulting from low dopaminergic input to the striatum are collectively called 'parkinsonism' and show that the basal ganglia are not correctly processing motor programmes. The signs are:
- Akinesia—poverty of movement, usually noticed first by lack of blinking and producing the characteristic expressionless face.
- Bradykinesia—when movement does occur it is very slow.
- Tremor at rest—with a frequency of 3–6 Hz. In the hands it is called a 'pill-rolling' tremor.
- Rigidity—caused by an increased tone in skeletal muscle. When passive movement is attempted the limbs move a little, then stop, then move again, then stop, etc. This is termed 'cog-wheel' rigidity.
- Micrographia—small handwriting results from inappropriate motor scaling.

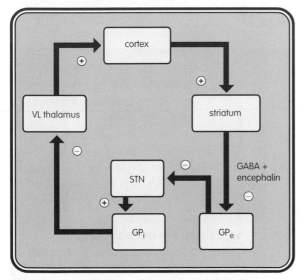

Fig. 4.16 The indirect loop. Striatal output inhibits the external globus pallidus (GP$_e$). This reduces the inhibition of the subthalamic nucleus (STN), and frees the STN to excite the internal globus pallidus (GP$_i$). Now the GP$_i$ can increase its inhibition of the cortex via the thalamus. (GABA, γ-aminobutyric acid; VL, ventrolateral.)

- Shuffling gait which increases in pace as walking distance increases, termed a 'festinating' gait.
- Abnormal postural reflexes producing a stooped, flexed posture.

The causes of the reduced nigrostriatal dopaminergic projection producing parkinsonism are:
- Parkinson's disease, an idiopathic condition where cells in the compact part of the substantia nigra which project to the striatum die, and so the dopaminergic input is lost. Other cell groups are also affected—the ventral tegmental area (dopamine to ventral striatum), locus ceruleus (noradrenaline projected diffusely in central nervous system) and the raphe nuclei (5-hydroxytryptamine projected diffusely in central nervous system).
- Postencephalitic parkinsonism.
- Neuroleptic medication taken for psychosis which antagonizes the dopamine input to the striatum.
- Neurotoxin ingestion, infamously by heroin addicts taking a synthetic morphine analogue contaminated with MPTP (1-methyl-4-phenyl-1,2,3,6-tetrahydropyridine). This is metabolized by monoamine oxidase B to a compound MPP⁺, which inhibits NADH dehydrogenase in dopaminergic terminals, reducing ATP production and promoting cell death.

The reductions in nigral cells producing parkinsonism are partly compensated for by:
- Increasing the number of dopamine receptors in the striatum.
- The remaining synapses releasing more dopamine (shown as an increase in the levels of dopamine metabolites compared with dopamine levels).

The signs of parkinsonism occur when the compensatory mechanisms fail, but this occurs only at 80% cell loss. Drug treatment of parkinsonism (here restricted to the treatment of Parkinson's disease) aims to increase the function of the remaining dopaminergic innervation to the striatum.

Anticholinergics (e.g. benzhexol and benztropine)
The arrangement of striatal circuitry (Fig. 4.14) shows that dopamine inhibits striatal output cells and acetylcholine excites them. To compensate for reduced dopamine input, acetylcholine antagonists can be given. Side effects are drowsiness, confusion (which can

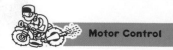

exacerbate dementia in Parkinson's disease), and reduced parasympathetic function. Acetylcholine is not the only excitatory input and this therapy will not work for long.

Dopamine precursors

This approach bypasses the rate-limiting step of dopamine synthesis—tyrosine hydroxylase. L-Dopa, the drug of choice for most Parkinson patients, is metabolized by dopa decarboxylase to dopamine.

Side effects of L-dopa are:

- Nausea and vomiting caused by stimulation of D_2 receptors in the chemoreceptor trigger zone in the brainstem.
- Reduction in gastric emptying due to effects on gastric dopamine receptors.
- Dyskinesias—the striatum becomes very sensitive to its dopamine input and overdose of L-dopa can occur producing involuntary movement.
- Psychiatric effects (psychosis, depression, toxic confusional state) due to alteration of all dopaminergic pathways that influence cortical function, e.g. ventral tegmental area to limbic system nuclei.

Side effects can be treated with a peripherally acting dopamine antagonist, domperidone, counteracting gastric emptying and nausea.

To increase the proportion of L-dopa reaching the central nervous system, drugs need to be given to prevent L-dopa from being utilized by peripheral nervous structures such as sympathetic nerve terminals. Carbidopa and benserazide are inhibitors of dopa decarboxylase that act only in the periphery, as they do not cross the blood–brain barrier, and are an essential addition to L-dopa therapy.

Long-term treatment (>5 years) does not prevent deterioration, akinesia recurs, equivalent doses give shorter periods of relief, and the response to L-dopa becomes unpredictable.

Inhibitors of monoamine oxidase B

Inhibitors of monoamine oxidase B, such as selegiline, reduce the rate at which dopamine is degraded in nerve terminals and potentiate the effect of L-dopa.

Direct dopamine agonists

Direct dopamine agonists (e.g. bromocriptine) stimulate striatal receptors but do not mimic the normal

conditions of dopamine release in the striatum. Side effects are similar to those of L-dopa—nausea and psychiatric disturbance.

Huntington's disease

This condition is caused by selective cell death in the striatum of acetylcholine neurons and GABA neurons. Hyperkinesia develops with squirming dance-like or 'choreic' movement. This is because initially GABAergic output cells projecting to the external globus pallidus die, releasing it from inhibition and resulting in greater inhibition at the next set of cells in the group—the subthalamic nucleus (subthalamic lesions by themselves produce contralateral involuntary movement).

Cognitive functions also deteriorate as striatal cell death continues, affecting the processing loops with the frontal lobes.

- Discuss the arrangement of the basal ganglia and the types of information carried in the input pathways and output pathways.
- Describe the basic arrangement of thalamic nuclei and how they are connected with the basal ganglia and cortex.
- What are the connections producing two cortical re-entrant loops through the basal ganglia? What is the function of this loop in terms of motor and cognitive function?
- What are the signs of parkinsonism, the causes of low dopamine input to the striatum, and the treatment of Parkinson's disease?
- Outline the effects of disease in the basal ganglia.

THE CEREBELLUM

Anatomy

The cerebellum is divided into four functional areas—the flocculonodular lobe, the vermis, and the intermediate and lateral parts of the cerebellar hemispheres.

There are three functional units—the flocculonodular lobe (vestibulocerebellum), the vermis with the intermediate part of the hemisphere (spinocerebellum), and the lateral part of the hemisphere (cerebrocerebellum).

Fig. 4.17 shows the divisions of the cerebellum including the deep nuclei that integrate cerebellar cortical processing, forming an output that passes through the superior cerebellar peduncle.

Fig. 4.18 shows the folding of the cerebellar cortex into lobules and folia which give the cerebellum its furrowed appearance.

Figs 4.19 and 4.20 show the inputs to and outputs from the cerebellum.

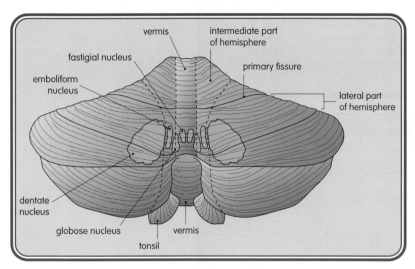

Fig. 4.17 The cerebellum (from the posterior aspect) showing nuclei lying deep within the cerebellum.

The cerebellar cortex

The processing circuit in the cerebellar cortex, as shown in Fig. 4.21, can be divided into input axons, processing interneurons, and output neurons.

Mossy fibres from the spinocerebellar tract, the dorsal column nuclei, and the pontocerebellar tract form the inputs, terminating on granule cells. Inputs from the inferior olivary nucleus in the brainstem (information from the spino-olivary tract, brainstem, and cortex) enter the circuit as climbing fibres and make many contacts on Purkinje cells.

The interneurons in the circuit have different functions.

- Granule cells, which receive most of the input to the cortex from the mossy fibres, send axons up towards the cortical surface, branching in parallel and making many contacts with other cell types in the cortical circuit.
- Golgi cells, after receiving excitation from granule cells, inhibit them.

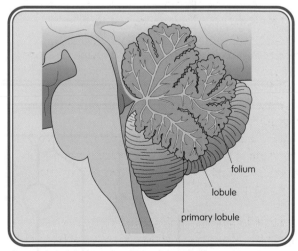

Fig. 4.18 Sagittal section through cerebellar cortex showing lobules and folia.

- Basket cells are also inhibitory and inhibit the output cell of the circuit—the Purkinje cell.

Routes of input to the cerebellum			
Origin and tract	**Peduncle**	**Termination**	**Processing**
spinal cord, anterior spinocerebellar	superior	vermis and paravermis	central pattern generator in walking
spinal cord, posterior spinocerebellar	inferior	vermis and paravermis	sensory
medulla, cuneocerebellar and gracilocerebellar, trigeminocerebellar	inferior	vermis and paravermis	sensory
midbrain, tectocerebellar	inferior	vermis	visual, auditory
medulla, olivocerebellar	inferior	paravermis	sensory
medulla, vestibulocerebellar	inferior	vermis and flocculus	balance
pons, pontocerebellar	middle	hemispheres	motor planning

Fig. 4.19 Routes of input to the cerebellum.

Cerebellar output			
Region	**Via deep nucleus**	**Termination**	**Function**
vermis	fastigial	motor cortex, reticular formation	control of axial muscles as movement progresses
paravermis	interposed	red nucleus—influencing fibres to thalamus and motor cortex, and those in rubrospinal tract	control of distal muscles as movement progresses
hemispheres	dentate	red nucleus and premotor cortex	movement planning, timing, and initiation
flocculonodular lobe	direct projection	lateral vestibular nucleus	control of balance and postural reflexes

Fig. 4.20 Cerebellar output.

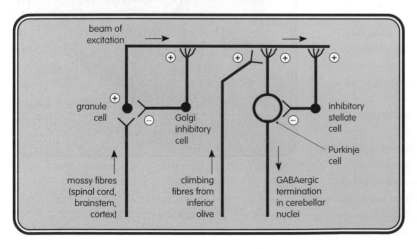

Fig. 4.21 The cerebellar cortex processing circuit.

The output of the circuit is from the Purkinje cell which also receives input from climbing fibres. Purkinje cells make GABAergic projections to the deep cerebellar nuclei which project to other parts of the central nervous system.

Functional units of the cerebellum

The vestibulocerebellum receives information from the vestibular nuclei (changes in head position relative to body position and gravity) and projects to the vestibular nuclei, lateral geniculate nuclei, superior colliculi, and striate cortex. It is involved in control of axial muscles (balance) and coordination of head and eye movements.

The spinocerebellum receives its main input from the spinocerebellar tract and is concerned with the control of muscle tone (by setting γ-motor neuron drive which affects α-motor neuron activity through the reflex loop) and movement execution.

- The vermis receives information from auditory, visual, and vestibular systems and sensory information from the proximal body. It projects to the motor cortex and reticular formation.
- The intermediate hemisphere receives sensory information from the distal body and projects through the red nucleus to the contralateral motor cortex.

The cerebrocerebellum controls precision in rapid and dextrous movements, receiving information from motor and sensory areas. It is inserted in a processing loop like the basal ganglia (motor cortex to pontine nuclei to cerebellar cortex to dentate nucleus to contralateral ventrolateral thalamic nucleus and red nucleus to motor cortex).

Error detection in cerebellar movement control

The Purkinje cells show an alteration in their firing pattern when errors in planned movement occur. This change consists of 'complex' spikes where, after the initial depolarization from the incoming Na^+, there is a smaller continued depolarization, a 'plateau' caused by incoming Ca^{2+}, and then further spikes superimposed on the plateau, again because of the opening of Ca^{2+} channels. This pattern of firing is produced by climbing fibre input and shows that the role of the olivocerebellar tract is in error detection.

Effects of cerebellar lesions

Cerebellar disease produces disorders in limbs ipsilateral to the lesion; volitional movements are still present although defective.

Lesions can result from head injury, tumours, haemorrhage, ischaemia, and Friedreich's ataxia. The white matter pathways carrying the connections can be damaged in multiple sclerosis.

Effects include the following:

- Disturbances of posture—wide-base standing position, ataxic gait, nystagmus in flocculonodular damage.
- Disturbances of muscle tone (hypotonia) and axial and truncal control—in vermis and intermediate hemisphere damage.
- Disturbances in control of precision movements—delays in starting and stopping movements, tremor increasing in severity through a movement, disorders in movement timing so that movements become decomposed into their components, and poor coordination of similarly acting muscle groups, making rapidly alternating movements very difficult.

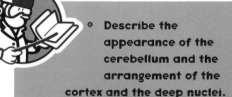

- Describe the appearance of the cerebellum and the arrangement of the cortex and the deep nuclei.
- Which cells form the circuitry in the cortex? What are their functions in input, processing, and output?
- The cerebellum needs different types of information for its role in motor control. Relate this to the sites of origin and termination of the anatomical pathways entering and leaving the cerebellum.
- What are the functions of the cerebellum? Relate them to the effects of lesions.

THE VESTIBULAR SYSTEM, POSTURE, AND LOCOMOTION

Control of posture

Posture

Posture is the relative position of the trunk, head and limbs in space. To keep posture stable, the body's centre of gravity needs to be maintained in position over its support base.

Postural reflexes are required to correct changes caused by displacement of the centre of gravity (by either external forces or deliberate movement). Postural change is detected by musculoskeletal proprioceptors, the vestibular apparatus, and the visual system.

The vestibular system

Fig. 4.22 shows the components of the vestibular system. The vestibular apparatus detects changes in head position, linear acceleration, and angular acceleration. The vestibular nuclei use this information together with afferent nerves from neck muscles and cervical vertebrae to determine if the head is moving alone or if the head and body are both moving. The nuclei can influence antigravity and axial musculature via a direct projection into the spinal cord.

The receptor system

Fig. 4.23 shows that the vestibular apparatus is composed of a number of interconnected membranous tunnels, collectively the membranous labyrinth, filled with a fluid called endolymph. The membranous labyrinth lies in a fluid-filled space in the temporal bone—the osseous labyrinth (as its margins are determined by bone)—and the fluid filling is termed perilymph.

Head movement is detected by movement of the membranous labyrinth relative to the endolymph which, because of its inertia, lags behind.

Specialized hair cells at certain points in the membranous labyrinths have projections from their surface into jelly-like masses floating in the endolymph.

The projections bend as the masses in the endolymph lag behind the movement of the labyrinth, as shown in Fig. 4.24. The membrane deformation produced alters the shape of cation channels and changes the membrane potential—depolarized for stereocilia bending towards the kinocilium, hyperpolarized if bent away.

The otolith organs lie in two areas of the membranous labyrinth—the saccule and utricle—which both contain patches of hair cells called maculae.

The projections from the surface of the hair cells lie in a jelly containing calcium salt crystals (the otoliths), as shown in Fig. 4.25. The otoliths have a higher specific weight than the endolymph, so the position of the otoliths relative to the maculae is influenced by gravity; this gives information about static head position, coded by slowly adapting receptors. Linear acceleration, coded by rapidly adapting receptors, is detected as the otoliths lag behind movement of the maculae.

The saccular otoliths are oriented vertically, and detect changes in linear acceleration in the vertical plane and changes in head position during lateral tilt.

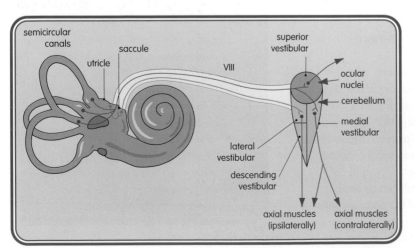

Fig. 4.22 The vestibular system.

The utricular otoliths are oriented horizontally, and detect changes in linear acceleration in the horizontal plane and changes in head position during flexion and extension of the neck.

The semicircular canals are arranged at right angles to each other and together they detect angular acceleration in all three planes of three-dimensional space.

Each canal has a swelling (ampulla) near its attachment to the utricle which contains the hair cells projecting from a ridge (crista) into a simple jelly-like substance (cupula) in the endolymph, as shown in Fig. 4.26.

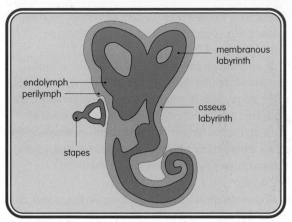

Fig. 4.23 Relationship between membranous and osseous labyrinths.

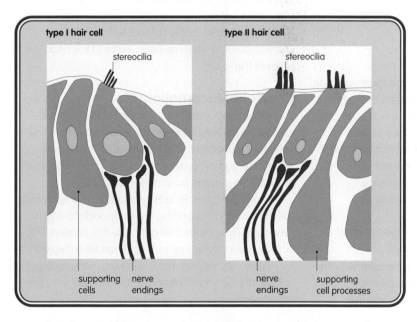

Fig. 4.24 Hair cells and afferent connections. There are two types of cochlear hair cells: type I (inner hair cells), which synapse with afferent nerve endings, and type II (outer hair cells) which synapse with efferent nerve endings.

Fig. 4.25 Structure of otolith organs.

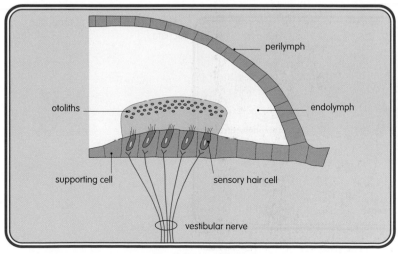

Improving the quality of postural information

Hair cells show greatest alteration in membrane permeability when the stereocilia are moved in one direction. To detect different degrees of tilt and different degrees of flexion, the hair cells in the maculae are oriented differently so that they respond best to a particular head position. The vestibular nuclei can use this information to assess head position precisely.

Complementary pathways

The brain receives complementary information from the labyrinths as they are located on opposite sides of the head. For example, as the head turns, one set of hair cells becomes depolarized, whereas the complementary set on the other side becomes hyperpolarized. This organization helps to mediate postural reflexes.

The vestibular nuclei

The vestibular nuclei lie in the floor of the fourth ventricle and receive information from the hair cells through the vestibular nerve (VIII). The semicircular canals project to the superior and medial nuclei; the otolith organs project to the lateral nuclei. The medial vestibulospinal tract projects bilaterally, and the lateral vestibulospinal tract projects ipsilaterally. Both tracts influence antigravity, axial, and limb extensor muscles.

Responses to external and self-generated disturbance

External disturbance alters the postural equilibrium. The vestibular system detects postural change and mediates postural adjustment. Together with the cerebellum, the vestibular system can adapt postural reflexes (e.g. responses on a moving platform as shown in Fig. 4.27).

Responses to self-generated disturbance show that the vestibular system has a feed-forward control mechanism. This is important for eye movements, as postural change will alter the position of a point of gaze on the retina (e.g. the horizontal vestibulo-ocular reflex where head movements are the stimulus for compensatory eye movements, as shown in Fig. 4.28).

The vestibulo-ocular reflex is an open loop reflex as it works without feedback. The cerebellum regulates the gain of the reflex (amount of eye movement to compensate for head movement).

Vestibular and neck reflexes

The vestibular system mediates some of the neck reflexes (Fig. 4.29).

Control of locomotion

Locomotion requires a coordination of the systems controlling posture and the systems producing voluntary movement. This ensures that the body is supported against gravity and that the centre of gravity lies over the support base during propulsion.

A rhythm of muscle activity is needed as each limb takes its turn in supporting the body and moving it forwards. The circuits that generate this pattern of activity are in the spinal cord and can be activated by higher centres (e.g. the brainstem). Sensory input is important in maintaining coordination of locomotion.

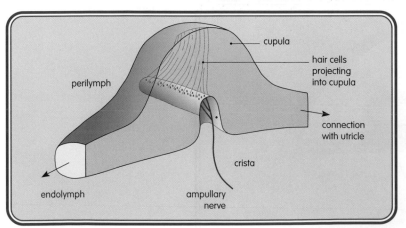

Fig. 4.26 Structure of ampullar crista.

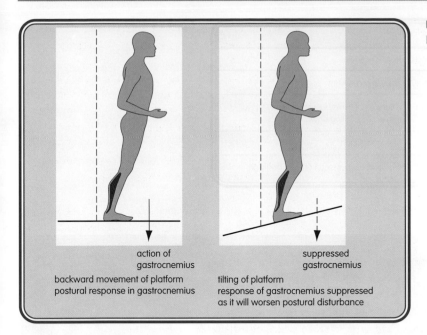

Fig. 4.27 Reflex responses to postural change can be altered.

action of
gastrocnemius

backward movement of platform
postural response in gastrocnemius

suppressed
gastrocnemius

tilting of platform
response of gastrocnemius suppressed
as it will worsen postural disturbance

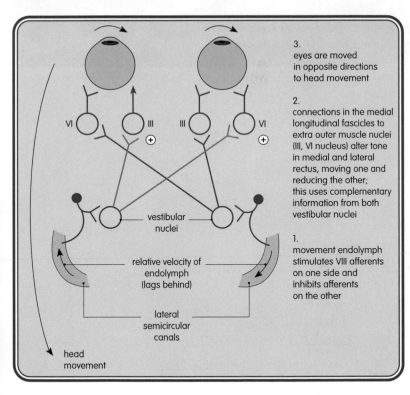

Fig. 4.28 The horizontal vestibulo-ocular reflex.

3.
eyes are moved
in opposite directions
to head movement

2.
connections in the medial
longitudinal fascicles to
extra outer muscle nuclei
(III, VI nucleus) alter tone
in medial and lateral
rectus, moving one and
reducing the other;
this uses complementary
information from both
vestibular nuclei

1.
movement endolymph
stimulates VIII afferents
on one side and
inhibits afferents
on the other

VI   III   III   VI

vestibular
nuclei

relative velocity of
endolymph
(lags behind)

lateral
semicircular
canals

head
movement

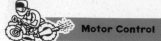
Fig. 4.29 Neck reflexes.

Neck reflexes		
Reflex	**Stimulus**	**Reflex action**
vestibulocollic	neck movement	oppose movement
vestibulospinal	falling (ventral tilting of head)	extension of arms, flexion of legs (protective if falling down)
cervicocollic	neck rotation	oppose rotation
cervicospinal	falling (ventral tilting of head)	flexion of arms, flexion of legs (partly protective)

○ **Name the components of the vestibular system.**
○ **What is the function of the otolith organs? Relate this to their response properties.**
○ **What is the function of the semicircular canals?**
○ **How does the vestibular system produce reflexes, such as the vestibulo-ocular reflex?**
○ **What is the function of the neck reflexes?**
○ **Describe the basic control of locomotion.**

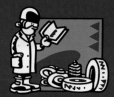

5. The Brainstem

THE BRAINSTEM NUCLEI

This section describes the anatomy of the brainstem by relating cross-sectional appearance to the overall structure of the brainstem.

Fig. 5.1 shows where the cranial nerves leave the brainstem and the levels of the seven brainstem sections shown in Figs 5.2–5.8. As you look through each cross-section, starting from the decussation of the pyramids upwards:

- Relate the site of exit of the cranial nerves to the connections with the nuclei in the brainstem.
- Relate the annotated functions of the nuclei with the distribution and function of the relevant cranial nerves.
- Note the variation in the cross-sectional appearance of the sensory tracts (formation of medial lemniscus) and motor tracts (formation of the pyramids) as they run through the brainstem.

- Discuss the organization of the brainstem nuclei as a continuation of the motor and sensory arrangement of the columns of cells in the spinal cord.
- Make labelled drawings of the cross-sectional appearances of different levels of the brainstem.
- Describe the arrangement and function of the cranial nerve nuclei.
- Summarize the crucial sensory role of the trigeminal nucleus as the relay station for all somatosensory information from the cranial nerves.

Fig. 5.1 Cranial nerves as they leave the brainstem.

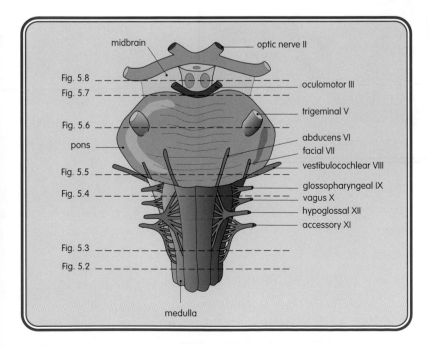

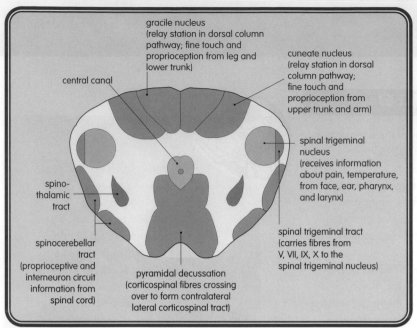

Fig. 5.2 Section through lower medulla.

gracile nucleus
(relay station in dorsal column pathway; fine touch and proprioception from leg and lower trunk)

cuneate nucleus
(relay station in dorsal column pathway; fine touch and proprioception from upper trunk and arm)

central canal

spinal trigeminal nucleus
(receives information about pain, temperature, from face, ear, pharynx, and larynx)

spino-thalamic tract

spinal trigeminal tract
(carries fibres from V, VII, IX, X to the spinal trigeminal nucleus)

spinocerebellar tract
(proprioceptive and interneuron circuit information from spinal cord)

pyramidal decussation
(corticospinal fibres crossing over to form contralateral lateral corticospinal tract)

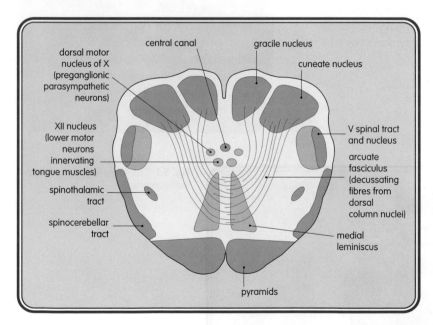

Fig. 5.3 Section through mid-medulla.

dorsal motor nucleus of X
(preganglionic parasympathetic neurons)

central canal

gracile nucleus

cuneate nucleus

XII nucleus
(lower motor neurons innervating tongue muscles)

V spinal tract and nucleus

arcuate fasciculus
(decussating fibres from dorsal column nuclei)

spinothalamic tract

spinocerebellar tract

medial leminiscus

pyramids

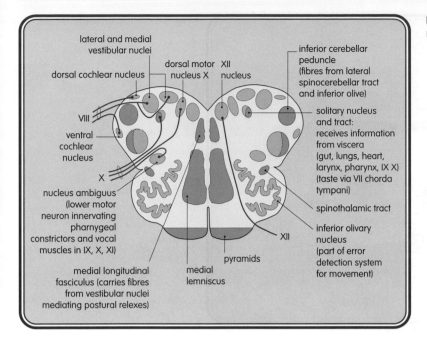

lateral and medial
vestibular nuclei

dorsal cochlear nucleus

dorsal motor
nucleus X

XII
nucleus

VIII

ventral
cochlear
nucleus

X

nucleus ambiguus
(lower motor
neuron innervating
pharnygeal
constrictors and vocal
muscles in IX, X, XI)

medial longitudinal
fasciculus (carries fibres
from vestibular nuclei
mediating postural relexes)

medial
lemniscus

pyramids

XII

inferior cerebellar
peduncle
(fibres from lateral
spinocerebellar tract
and inferior olive)

solitary nucleus
and tract:
receives information
from viscera
(gut, lungs, heart,
larynx, pharynx, IX X)
(taste via VII chorda
tympani)

spinothalamic tract

inferior olivary
nucleus
(part of error
detection system
for movement)

Fig. 5.4 Section through upper medulla.

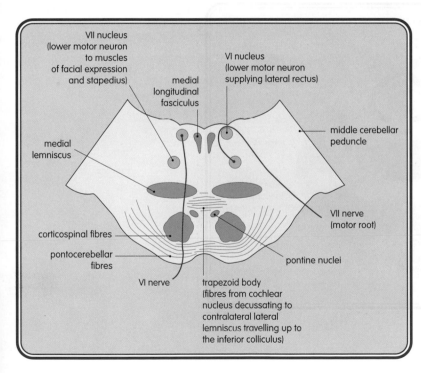

VII nucleus
(lower motor neuron
to muscles
of facial expression
and stapedius)

medial
longitudinal
fasciculus

VI nucleus
(lower motor neuron
supplying lateral rectus)

medial
lemniscus

middle cerebellar
peduncle

corticospinal fibres

pontocerebellar
fibres

VI nerve

trapezoid body
(fibres from cochlear
nucleus decussating to
contralateral lateral
lemniscus travelling up to
the inferior colliculus)

pontine nuclei

VII nerve
(motor root)

Fig. 5.5 Section through lower pons.

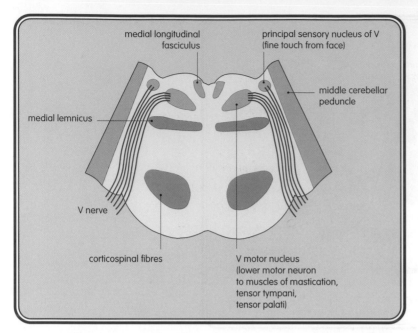

Fig. 5.6 Section through upper pons.

Labels on figure:
- medial longitudinal fasciculus
- principal sensory nucleus of V (fine touch from face)
- middle cerebellar peduncle
- medial lemnicus
- V nerve
- corticospinal fibres
- V motor nucleus (lower motor neuron to muscles of mastication, tensor tympani, tensor palati)

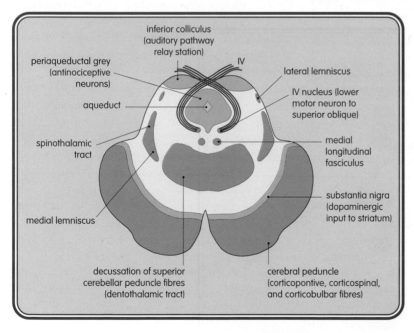

Fig. 5.7 Section through lower midbrain.

Labels on figure:
- inferior colliculus (auditory pathway relay station)
- IV
- periaqueductal grey (antinociceptive neurons)
- lateral lemniscus
- IV nucleus (lower motor neuron to superior oblique)
- aqueduct
- medial longitudinal fasciculus
- spinothalamic tract
- substantia nigra (dopaminergic input to striatum)
- medial lemniscus
- decussation of superior cerebellar peduncle fibres (dentothalamic tract)
- cerebral peduncle (corticopontine, corticospinal, and corticobulbar fibres)

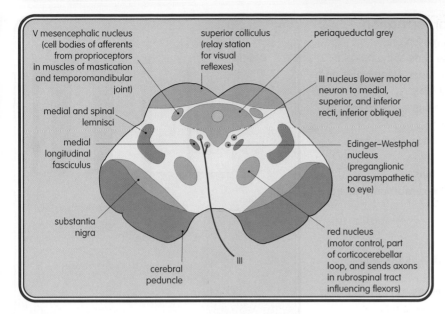

Fig. 5.8 Section through upper midbrain.

V mesencephalic nucleus (cell bodies of afferents from proprioceptors in muscles of mastication and temporomandibular joint)

superior colliculus (relay station for visual reflexes)

periaqueductal grey

III nucleus (lower motor neuron to medial, superior, and inferior recti, inferior oblique)

medial and spinal lemnisci

medial longitudinal fasciculus

Edinger–Westphal nucleus (preganglionic parasympathetic to eye)

substantia nigra

red nucleus (motor control, part of corticocerebellar loop, and sends axons in rubrospinal tract influencing flexors)

cerebral peduncle

III

THE RETICULAR FORMATION

Location and organization

If all the cell groups and tracts are identified in the brainstem (medulla, pons, and midbrain), one is left with a central core of cells arranged as a network and called, therefore, the brainstem reticular formation. It possibly represents a continuation of spinal cord interneurons.

In this central core, cell groupings can be identified on the basis of their containing a specific neurotransmitter. Four such groupings can be identified using noradrenaline, 5-hydroxytryptamine (5-HT), acetylcholine, and dopamine. These projections are extensive, with the exception of the dopaminergic system which projects to the striatal system, limbic areas, prefrontal cortex, and anterior cingulate cortex.

The remainder of the reticular core is, as yet, not separable in terms of chemical content but can be partially defined according to function. There is a

sensory portion in the lower medulla and lower pons (receiving spinoreticular fibres) and a motor portion in the upper medulla and upper pons (receiving fibres from the corticospinal tract giving rise to the reticulospinal tracts).

The pontine and medullary neurons project into the midbrain reticular formation which in turn projects mainly to the hypothalamus and also the thalamic reticular and intralaminar nuclei. There is also a large projection from the hypothalamus and prefrontal association cortex into the reticular formation.

The cells of the reticular formation can be histologically separated from other neurons, as shown in Fig. 5.9, in that:

- They have large laterally oriented dendritic trees which receive information from many sources.
- They project diffusely either to higher parts of the nervous system or to the spinal cord (most reticular cells have an upward and downward projection).

Fig. 5.9 A reticular formation neuron.

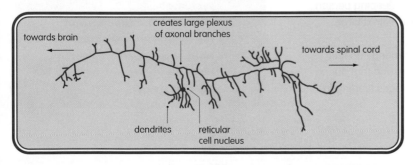

towards brain

creates large plexus of axonal branches

towards spinal cord

dendrites

reticular cell nucleus

Function of the reticular formation

The functions of the reticular formation are:

- Sleeping and waking—some parts of the reticular formation are involved in producing sleep states and others in awakening mechanisms.
- Behavioural arousal and awareness (particularly the noradrenergic system).
- Modulation of sensory information across the thalamic relay nuclei.
- Modulation of spinal interneurons.
- Transmitting information to the cerebellum—lateral parts of the reticular formation.
- Modulation of pain.
- Modulation of respiration.
- Modulation of responsiveness of hippocampal neurons.
- Integration of autonomic functions—in falling asleep, heart rate, blood pressure, and respiration all decline; before awakening, they are adjusted so that the transition from horizontal to vertical does not cause fainting.
- Possible role in cognition.
- Motor acts involving motivation and reward (dopaminergic system, particularly the mesolimbic projections from the midbrain to the ventral striatum).

Sleep and the electroencephalograph

The electroencephalograph (EEG) is a record of the electrical activity produced by the brain. It is obtained by attaching electrodes to the skull and connecting them to a suitable amplifier. In the awake subject, the frequency content of the EEG is mainly of frequencies above 20 Hz.

As one progresses into drowsiness and then to deep sleep, the frequency content decreases below 10 Hz (i.e. the waves recorded from the skull become slower).

Phases of paradoxical sleep or rapid eye movement (REM) sleep occur in which the EEG is of the awake pattern but the muscles of the neck are silent. This phase of sleep is important because a sleeping person woken in this phase will report dreams with a large content of visual imagery.

Fig. 5.10 shows that sleep can be divided into four phases according to the EEG frequency and that during sleep we cycle through the different stages tending to awaken just after a REM phase.

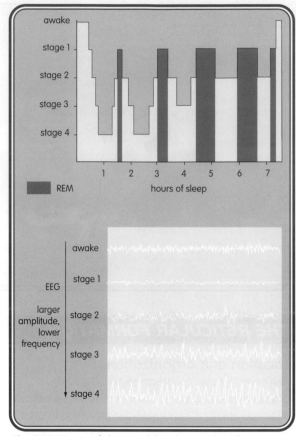

Fig. 5.10 Stages of sleep and the sleep cycle with electroencephalographs.

- Describe the anatomy of the reticular formation.
- How can this network be divided into neurochemical systems?
- What are the functions of the reticular formation?
- Name the stages of sleep. How does reticular activity control sleep?

BRAINSTEM-ACTING DRUGS AND GENERAL ANAESTHETICS

Nausea and vomiting
The vomiting response consists of:
- Reverse peristalsis, where the contents of the duodenum and jejunum are propelled back into the stomach.
- Closure of the glottis.
- Relaxation of the lower oesophageal sphincter.
- Contraction of the muscles of the abdominal wall.

These events, together with the sensation of nausea, are coordinated by an area in the medulla, the vomiting centre, which sends outputs to the dorsal motor nucleus of cranial nerve X and to the spinal motor neurons innervating the abdominal musculature. The types of stimuli that produce a vomiting response are explained by the inputs to the vomiting centre.

The chemoreceptor trigger zone in the area postrema in the medulla senses information about circulating compounds as it is not protected by the blood–brain barrier. Its neural circuits have many receptors (e.g. D_2, 5-HT_3, opioid) that allow pharmacological intervention to reduce information flow about chemical triggers. Drugs inducing nausea include L-dopa, opioids, anticancer agents (e.g. cisplatin), digitalis, and anaesthetics.

The vestibular system sends balance information to the vomiting centre. In motion sickness (pallor, sweating, nausea, and vomiting) there is a conflict between the visual and vestibular systems; this can be treated behaviourally or with drugs that reduce vestibular input. Vestibular disease presents with vertigo (false sense of rotary movement), particularly in labyrinthitis (seen acutely in viral infection—vertigo, nausea, and vomiting) and in Ménière's disease (vertigo, nausea, vomiting, tinnitus, and deafness) produced by increased endolymphatic pressure.

The solitary nucleus sends viscerosensory information about chemicals in the gut collected by cranial nerve X. The enteroendocrine system in the gut wall responds to gut contents and by 5-HT mechanisms can affect the firing of cranial nerve X afferent neurons.

The spinal cord sends information about trauma: nausea can accompany physical injury.

The limbic cortex sends information from the special senses: certain odours and sights can cause nausea.

Fig. 5.11 summarizes the connections of the medullary vomiting centre and the sites of drug action.

Antiemetics
Fig. 5.12 shows the action, uses, and side effects of some antiemetic drugs.

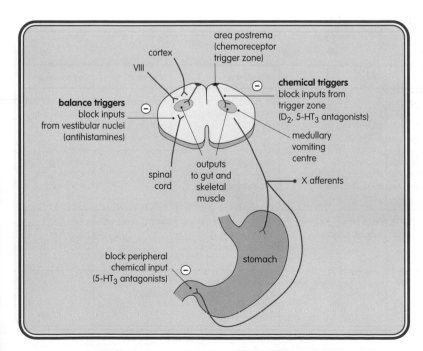

Fig. 5.11 Sites of action of antiemetics.

cortex
VIII
area postrema (chemoreceptor trigger zone)
chemical triggers block inputs from trigger zone (D_2, 5-HT_3 antagonists)
balance triggers block inputs from vestibular nuclei (antihistamines)
medullary vomiting centre
spinal cord
outputs to gut and skeletal muscle
X afferents
block peripheral chemical input (5-HT_3 antagonists)
stomach

Antiemetic drugs				
Class	Drug	Site of action	Uses	Side effects
antimuscarinic	hyoscine	vomiting centre, antagonizing vestibular input	motion sickness	drowsiness, dry mouth, blurred vision, impaired short-term memory
antihistamine	cinnarizine and cyclizine	vomiting centre, antagonizing vestibular input	motion sickness, vestibular disease	less than antihistamines
other	betahistine	reduces endolymphatic pressure in the membranous labyrinths	Meniere's disease	
D_2 antagonists	metoclopramide and domperidone	chemoreceptor trigger zone reducing sensitivity to chemical triggers in the blood	reduces drug-induced nausea and vomiting; combination with paracetamol to treat migraine	drowsiness, fatigue, motor restlessness
$5-HT_3$ antagonist	ondansetron and granisetron	chemoreceptor trigger zone and peripherally in the gut reducing transmission from 5-HTergic enteroendocrine cells in response to chemical triggers in the gut	reduces drug-induced nausea and vomiting	headache, gastrointestinal upset
atypical	dexamethasone	unknown mechanism of action; pharmacologically it is a glucocorticoid	taken in combination with ondansetron to reduce drug-induced nausea and vomiting	side effects seen after long-term high-dose regime

Fig. 5.12 Antiemetic drugs.

Drugs acting on brainstem monoaminergic systems

The brainstem monoaminergic systems project into the thalamus and cortex with a rather diffuse innervation. This is because these systems have a general modulatory function. Drugs acting on these systems are usually self-administered as drugs of abuse because of their effects on monoaminergic systems that modulate processing of thought and emotion (Fig. 5.13).

General anaesthesia

All general anaesthetic agents produce:

Drugs of abuse						
Class	Drug	Action	Effects	Side effects	Tolerance	Dependence
psychomotor stimulants	amphetamine	causes release of NA and DA from terminals	central DA effects: euphoria, excitement, locomotor stimulation with repetitive behaviour (stereotypies), anorexia; peripheral NA effects: increased blood pressure, decreased gastrointestinal motility	insomnia, irritability, headache, psychosis, tremor	develops as amphetamine depletes terminals of transmitter	increases activity in DA reward system (VTA to nucleus acumbens), producing psychological dependence
	cocaine	blocks NA and DA uptake (uptake 1)		cardiac dysrhythmias, convulsions, respiratory and vasomotor depression		
hallucinogens	lysergic acid diethylamide (LSD)	$5-HT_2$ partial agonist	altered perception, thoughts, feelings	persistent effects lasting several weeks, flashbacks to previous 'trips'	quickly develops	none
	MDMA (Ecstasy)	amphetamine-like and LSD-like	euphoria and altered thoughts	idiosyncratic responses—coma, convulsions, hyperpyrexia, rhabdomyolysis	cross tolerance with LSD	none

Fig. 5.13 Drugs of abuse. (DA, dopamine; NA, noradrenaline; VTA, ventral tegmental area.)

- Loss of consciousness, of reflex responses to noxious stimuli, of spatial orientation, of volitional control, and of memory, and reductions in respiratory rate and blood pressure.
- Death at high doses, caused by respiratory depression and cardiovascular depression by actions on the medulla; also, cardiac depression may be brought about by direct effects on the myocardium.

Anaesthesia used to be characterized by an initial excitatory phase (modern anaesthetics act very quickly so that this phase is no longer prolonged or troublesome) followed by a dose-dependent increase in anaesthetic depth.

There is no obvious pharmacological structure–activity relationship for anaesthetic agents; their mechanisms of action are complex, either by affecting the reticular formation (most anaesthetics) or by a direct depression of cortical activity (e.g. propofol).

The potency of any anaesthetic is directly related to its hydrophobic nature, generally measured as its lipid solubility as the oil:gas (for gases and vapours) and oil:water (for aqueous agents) partition coefficient. One possible mechanism of action is that anaesthetics interact with a hydrophobic region (either lipid, protein, or lipoprotein) of the neuronal membrane, causing membrane expansion and consequent malfunction. Evidence for this is that anaesthesia in mammals may be reversed by high ambient pressure (in excess of 100 atm; 10.1 MPa).

Induction and recovery

Induction and recovery describe how quickly anaesthesia occurs after administration and how quickly the body recovers from anaesthesia. The speed of induction with and recovery from an anaesthetic depend upon the physical properties of the anaesthetic and how quickly it can equilibrate between the lungs, blood, and central nervous system for inhalants and gaseous agents or from blood and central nervous system for aqueous agents.

After equilibration, 95% of the administered anaesthetic is in the body fat. Fat has a low blood flow and so it takes a long time for anaesthetics to enter and leave the body fat—a very fat-soluble anaesthetic can build up gradually in adipose tissue and then be released back into the circulation over a long period of time.

The most common general anaesthetics are compared in Fig. 5.14.

Anaesthetic drugs				
Route	Drug	Potency (oil:gas)	Induction/recovery	Notes and side effects
inhaled	N_2O	low (1.4)	fast	Only analgesic by itself. Used 60%O_2/40% N_2O as carrier for other agents
	halothane	high (220)	medium	Depresses myocardium, baroreceptor reflex, sympathetic system producing hypotension. 20% metabolized and may cause hepatic damage
	enflurane	medium (98)	medium	Depresses myocardium producing hypotension. 2% metabolized so no hepatic damage. May cause seizures
	isoflurane	medium (91)	medium	Causes vasodilatation producing hypotension. Only 0.2% metabolized. Less epileptogenic than enflurane but may cause myocardial ischaemia
injected	thiopentone	high	fast	Depresses myocardium and respiratory centre. Not analgesic. 12–16% of dose metabolized per hour. Short duration of action as redistributed in body fat
	propofol		fast	Cardiovascular and respiratory depression. Rapidly metabolized and suitable for total intravenous anaesthesia

Fig. 5.14 Anaesthetic drugs.

- Describe the vomiting response in relation to the inputs and outputs of the vomiting centre.
- State the actions, uses, and side effects of common antiemetics.
- Discuss the function of monoaminergic inputs to the cortex from the brainstem and how drugs acting on these systems are used as drugs of abuse.
- Summarize the principles of general anaesthetic action in relation to lipid solubility. State the effects and side effects of the common agents.

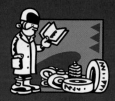

6. The Autonomic Nervous System

INTRODUCTION

As a general principle, the autonomic nervous system controls the supply of nutrients, the removal of waste products, and the distribution of the blood supply.

The control of these processes is involuntary, widespread, and relatively slow, aimed at the visceral organs, and depends on the output of the three divisions of the autonomic nervous system—the sympathetic, parasympathetic, and enteric nervous systems.

These systems are controlled and integrated by the hypothalamus (which influences preganglionic neurons of the sympathetic and parasympathetic systems) and the nucleus of the solitary tract (which integrates sensory inflow and output of the autonomic divisions of the cranial nerve nuclei).

STRUCTURE AND FUNCTION OF THE SYMPATHETIC NERVOUS SYSTEM

Physiological role of the sympathetic nervous system

The sympathetic system prepares the body for responses to stressful challenges, condensed into the sequence 'flight, fright, or fight', allowing sudden strenuous exercise and increased vigilance.

The sympathetic nervous system also helps control blood pressure, thermoregulation, gut function, and urogenital function.

Structure of the sympathetic nervous system

A column of cells (intermediolateral column) runs from T1 to L2 and contains the cell bodies of neurons whose axons contact a chain of ganglia outside the central nervous system lying along the vertebral column (paravertebral ganglia), as shown in Fig. 6.1.

Preganglionic neurons send axons through the ventral root of their segmental spinal nerve to the ganglia and synapse on neurons that innervate target organs.

Each preganglionic neuron can influence many neurons in different ganglia by collaterals, coordinating

the activation of ganglia at different spinal levels, as seen in Fig. 6.2.

Postganglionic axons are unmyelinated and pass into peripheral nerves to target sites. For the head and neck, they form a plexus around the carotid arteries and gain access to the interior of the skull by the internal carotid artery.

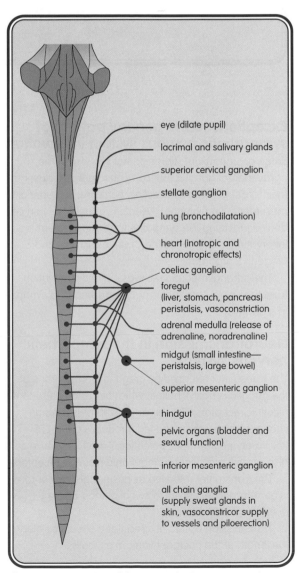

eye (dilate pupil)

lacrimal and salivary glands

superior cervical ganglion

stellate ganglion

lung (bronchodilatation)

heart (inotropic and chronotropic effects)

coeliac ganglion

foregut (liver, stomach, pancreas) peristalsis, vasoconstriction

adrenal medulla (release of adrenaline, noradrenaline)

midgut (small intestine—peristalsis, large bowel)

superior mesenteric ganglion

hindgut

pelvic organs (bladder and sexual function)

inferior mesenteric ganglion

all chain ganglia (supply sweat glands in skin, vasoconstricor supply to vessels and piloerection)

Fig. 6.1 Organization of the sympathetic nervous system.

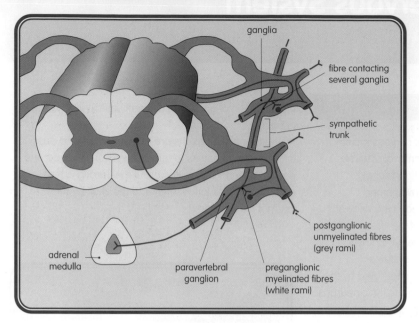

Fig. 6.2 Spinal cord efferents to the sympathetic chain.

Exceptions to the general pattern of sympathetic nervous system innervation

Some postganglionic fibres do not synapse in the paravertebral ganglia, but carry on to ganglia closer to their target organs. The coeliac, aorticorenal, superior mesenteric, and inferior mesenteric ganglia contain cell bodies providing the sympathetic nervous system innervation to the gut, kidney, liver, pancreas, and urogenital organs.

The adrenal medulla receives a direct innervation from the spinal cord that is not interrupted by a synapse in a ganglion.

Neurotransmission in the sympathetic nervous system

The transmitter released by preganglionic neurons at the ganglia is acetylcholine, which binds to postsynaptic nicotinic receptors. The nicotinic receptor is a cation channel which, when opened, produces a fast EPSP (excitatory postsynaptic potential). Adrenal medulla cells also receive a cholinergic input onto nicotinic receptors.

The transmitter released by postganglionic neurons is noradrenaline, except in sweat glands where acetylcholine is released.

Transmission occurs at specialized structures along the length of the postganglionic axon, called varicosities, which synthesize, release, take up, and metabolize noradrenaline. This process is called *en passage* transmission—the action potential does not end when noradrenaline is released but carries on to the next varicosity.

Cells of the adrenal medulla release noradrenaline and adrenaline into the circulation, permitting the sympathetic nervous system to have a general humoral action on adrenergic receptors in the body.

The effect of noradrenaline release is dependent on the type of receptor that is present in the target organ, as shown in Fig. 6.3. Sweat glands have muscarinic receptors that bind the released acetylcholine.

Other transmitters

Often, cotransmitters are released with the main transmitter in the sympathetic nervous system and have a longer-lasting and more subtle modulatory influence on postsynaptic activity (e.g. neuropeptide Y and vasoactive intestinal polypeptide).

Drugs acting on the sympathetic nervous system
The ganglia

Drugs affecting ganglionic transmission have no clinical use. They have complex actions because parasympathetic and sympathetic postganglionic neurons are influenced at the same time, often with opposing effects. Agonists at ganglionic nicotinic receptors (e.g. nicotine) produce hypertension and tachycardia. Antagonists (e.g. hexamethonium) produce hypotension, but cannot be used as antihypertensive agents because of their side-effect profile.

Target organs

Noradrenergic transmission can be altered by interfering with noradrenaline synthesis, release, or postsynaptic interaction with different receptor subtypes. Drugs used clinically are shown in Fig. 6.4.

- What is the role of the sympathetic nervous system and how does this relate to its structure and pattern of innervation?
- State the clinical uses of drugs that act on the sympathetic nervous system.

Adrenergic receptors			
Adrenergic receptor	**Location**	**Second messenger**	**Function**
α_1	smooth muscle in blood vessels and bronchi, dilator pupillae	IP_3	contraction
α_2	smooth muscle in blood vessels, presynaptically on adrenergic synapses	decreased cAMP	contraction, reduced transmitter release
β_1	heart muscle, presynaptically on adrenergic synapses	increased cAMP	increased heart rate and force of contraction, increased transmitter release
β_2	smooth muscle in blood vessels and bronchi	decreased cAMP	relaxation

Fig. 6.3 Adrenergic receptors: location, second messenger, and function.

Drugs acting on the sympathetic nervous system			
Drug	**Action**	**Clinical use**	**Side effects**
adrenaline	α, β agonist	anaphylaxis, cardiac arrest	hypertension, dysrhythmia
salbutamol	β_2 agonist	asthma	tachycardia, dysrhythmia, tremor
clonidine	partial α_2 agonist	hypertension	drowsiness, postural hypotension
prazosin	α_1 antagonist	hypertension	hypotension, tachycardia, impotence
atenolol	β_1 antagonist	hypertension, angina, dysrhythmia	heart failure, fatigue, cold extremities, less bronchoconstriction than non-selective β antagonists

Fig. 6.4 Drugs acting on the sympathetic nervous system.

STRUCTURE AND FUNCTION OF THE PARASYMPATHETIC NERVOUS SYSTEM

Physiological role of the parasympathetic nervous system

The parasympathetic nervous system has many actions, which can be described as:

- Opposing some effects of the sympathetic nervous system (heart rate, gut motility, and bronchiolar diameter).
- Controlling body functions under non-stressful conditions, working either alone or with the sympathetic nervous system (e.g. ciliary muscle for accommodation for near objects; gastrointestinal secretions; secretions of the nose, mouth, and eye; micturition; defaecation; sexual function).

Structure of the parasympathetic nervous system

There are two clusters of preganglionic neurons at either end of the spinal cord. The cranial parasympathetic nervous system outflow comes from several nuclei in the brainstem, whose neurons travel in cranial nerves to reach the appropriate ganglion and then (sometimes in a different cranial nerve) to reach the target organ. The sacral parasympathetic nervous system outflow comes from preganglionic neurons whose cell bodies lie in a column running from segments S2 to S4 of the spinal cord, with their axons leaving the cord through the ventral root.

The ganglia lie much closer to their target organs than those of the sympathetic nervous system, as shown in Fig. 6.5.

Neurotransmission in the parasympathetic nervous system

At the ganglia, like the sympathetic nervous system, preganglionic neurons release acetylcholine onto postsynaptic nicotinic receptors.

At target organs, postganglionic neurons release acetylcholine onto muscarinic receptors, which show subtype variation localized to different target organs (Fig. 6.6).

Drugs acting on the parasympathetic nervous system

The drugs in clinical use that affect the function of the parasympathetic nervous system interact with the receptors on the target organs (Fig. 6.7).

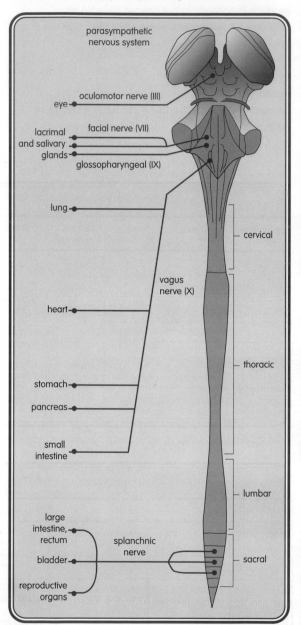

Fig. 6.5 Organization of the parasympathetic nervous system.

THE ENTERIC NERVOUS SYSTEM

The enteric nervous system is a neural system embedded in the wall of the alimentary tract, pancreas, and gall bladder. It consists of two tubular systems—the myenteric (Auerbach's) and submucous (Meissner's) plexuses—containing sensory neurons and motor neurons as well as interneurons.

The sensory neurons monitor the mechanical state of the alimentary canal, the chemical status of the stomach and intestinal contents, and the hormonal levels in the blood.

The output motor neurons control gut motility and secretion as well as the diameter of local blood vessels.

The parasympathetic nervous system and sympathetic nervous system can override the enteric division.

- ○ **What is the role of the parasympathetic nervous system and how is this related to its structure and pattern of innervation?**
- ○ **Compare the innervation pattern and structure with that of the sympathetic nervous system.**
- ○ **What are the clinical uses of drugs that alter the function of the parasympathetic nervous system?**
- ○ **Describe the structure and function of the enteric nervous system.**

Drugs acting on the parasympathetic nervous system			
Muscarinic subtype	**Location**	**Second messenger and postsynaptic effect**	**Function**
M_1	gastric parietal cells, enteric nervous system	increased IP_3, producing slow EPSP	gastric acid secretion, gastrointestinal motility
M_2	cardiac atrium	decreased cAMP, producing slow EPSP	reducing heart rate
M_3	smooth muscle, glands	increased IP_3 causing increased intracellular Ca^{2+}	secretion, smooth muscle contraction

Fig. 6.6 Drugs acting on the parasympathetic nervous system.

Muscarinic receptors			
Drug	**Action**	**Use**	**Side effects**
pilocarpine	Partial muscarinic agonist	glaucoma (increased intraocular pressure), where increased constrictor pupillae action allows greater drainage of aqueous humour	cardiac slowing, increased gastrointestinal tract activity causing abdominal pain
bethanechol	muscarinic agonist	rarely used for stimulating bladder emptying	as for pilocarpine
atropine	muscarinic antagonist	sinus bradycardia after myocardial infarction	dry mouth, dilated pupil, blurred vision, bronchodilatation, urinary retention
ipratropium	muscarinic antagonist	asthma, causing bronchodilatation and inhibiting increases in mucous secretion	inhaled and does not pass easily into the circulation, so few side effects
dicyclomine	M_1 antagonist has direct relaxant effect on smooth muscle	reduce spasmodic activity of gastrointestinal tract in irritable bowel syndrome	less severe than atropine
pirenzipine	M_1 antagonist	peptic ulcer, reducing gastric acid secretion	no marked side effects

Fig. 6.7 Muscarinic receptors.

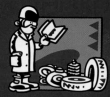

7. Vision

THE EYE

Anatomy of the eye—transparent structures

The structures inside the eye are shown in Fig. 7.1.
The cornea consists of five layers.

- An epithelial layer of stratified squamous cells is richly innervated with sensory nerves; it rests on a basement membrane.
- The basement membrane gives strength to the cornea; it rests on the corneal stroma.
- The corneal stroma occupies 90% of the thickness of the cornea. It consists of thin sheets of collagen fibrils that are oriented parallel to each other in the same sheet and at right angles to fibrils in sheets either side. The spacing and arrangement of the fibrils gives the cornea its transparency.
- A basal lamina lines the inner surface of the stroma, forming the base for the endothelial layer.
- The endothelial layer is a single layer of squamous cells providing mechanisms for metabolic exchange between the aqueous humour and the cornea. It regulates the water content of the corneal stroma, preventing oedema and consequent opacity.

The lens consists of three parts:

- It is encapsulated in a basement membrane that is elastic, and strongest at the insertion of the suspensory ligament around the equator of the lens.
- Lining the inside of the capsule on its anterior surface is a layer of cuboidal cells (subcapsular epithelium). Epithelial cells near the lateral equator differentiate into lens fibres.
- Lens fibres are thin, flattened, and devoid of organelles and nuclei. They become filled with proteins (crystallins) and extend towards the centre of the lens, producing a very dense central section.

The lens changes with age. It loses its ability to accommodate as its elasticity reduces. It loses its transparency because of changes in proteins in the fibres. Opacity can also be produced if the lens becomes dehydrated (cataract formation).

The shape of the eye is maintained by the tough sclera and an internal pressure (the intraocular pressure) exerted by the aqueous humour, which is formed by ultrafiltration in the ciliary body and drained through the scleral sinus.

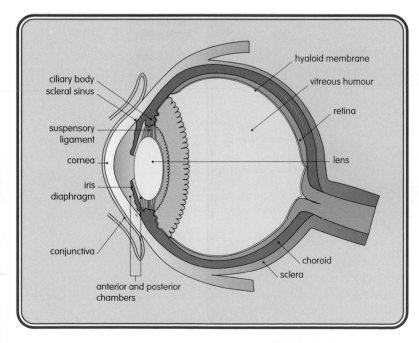

Fig. 7.1 Cross-section through the eye showing the main structures.

hyaloid membrane

vitreous humour

retina

ciliary body
scleral sinus

suspensory ligament

cornea

lens

iris
diaphragm

conjunctiva

choroid

sclera

anterior and posterior chambers

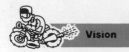

The normal intraocular pressure is usually 10–20 mmHg; if it exceeds 22 mmHg, the condition of glaucoma is produced, which can produce blindness by compressing the blood supply to the optic nerve. Blockages in the scleral sinus (e.g. by drugs which dilate the pupil, thereby constricting the connective-tissue network of the sinus) can cause sharp rises in intraocular pressure.

The eye is adapted for acute vision by having one small area of its sensory layer containing a vast number of photoreceptors (specifically for colour vision in good illumination), which it can direct accurately and quickly to different areas of space.

This central area is the fovea lying 3 mm lateral to the optic disc as shown in Fig. 7.2, and it differs from the rest of the retina because:

- Only cone receptors are present at a very high density.
- It has no overlying vascular network.
- Overlying neural elements are displaced to allow maximal light access.

The fovea is the central part of a small circular region called the macula lutea. On examination with an ophthalmoscope, the pigmented epithelium underlying the macula shows through, giving it a darker appearance than the rest of the retina.

Optics of the eye

Light from a point of visual fixation is bent (refracted) so that a clearly focused image appears on the retina (Fig. 7.3). The lens for the visual system is a compound lens with interfaces of different refractive power (measured in dioptres, D) at the cornea, between the anterior chamber and the lens, and between the lens and the vitreous body. The total refractive power is 58.6 D, with most of the power (42 D) at the air–cornea interface.

The refractive power of the lens is changed by accommodation. When the ciliary muscle contracts it moves downwards and forwards, reducing the tension in the suspensory ligament and allowing the elastic lens to become fatter and shorter, so that it focuses light from near targets onto the retina.

The clarity of the focused image is increased by pupillary constriction. This is because reduction in pupil diameter allows light to pass through only the centre of the lens, where spherical aberration is at its lowest; thus pupillary constriction occurs via a reflex pathway during accommodation.

The visual axis of the eye does not correspond to its geometrical axis and is displaced so that the visual axis runs through the fovea (Fig. 7.4).

The retina responds to a restricted range of wavelengths of light. We see and perceive colours in

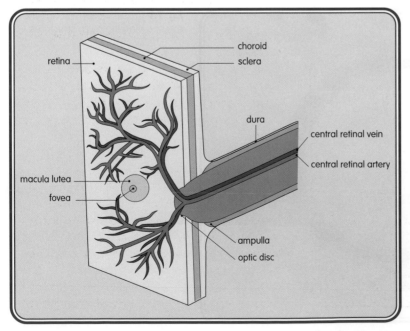

Fig. 7.2 Section of retina containing the fundus.

the range 400 nm (violet) to 780 nm (red). Wavelengths either side of this range (as low as 400 nm and as high as 1400 nm) penetrate the eye, but are not perceived.

The cornea and lens become yellow with age and this filters out a lot of light in the blue wavelength band.

○ **Describe the functions of the different structures in the eyeball in relation to structural support, nutritional support, transparency, refraction, and receptor function.**

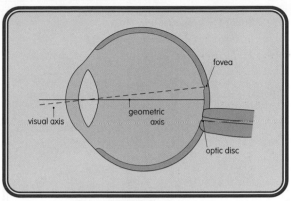

Fig. 7.4 Visual axis of the eye.

RETINAL FUNCTION AND IMAGE PROCESSING

Structure of the retina

The neural part of the retina responds to light, processes light signals from photoreceptors, and sends visual information to the thalamus and brainstem. The functions of different neurons in the retina depend on their connections and all the neural elements are supported with a type of glial cell, Müller's cell.

There is a blood–retina barrier at the endothelium of the capillary network on the anterior surface of the retina, from the central retinal artery, and at the endothelium of the capillary network in the choroid.

The receptor function of the retina is carried out by two types of cell:

- Rods are very sensitive and respond to dim light and are found peripherally in the retina.
- Cones are less sensitive and respond best in bright light. There are three types of cones differentiated by their response to light of different wavelengths and they are clustered in the fovea, where the visual axis meets the retina.

Rods and cones have different structures, as shown in Figs 7.5 and 7.6, but share the following features:

- Outer segments, which contact the pigmented epithelial layer of the retina, contain highly folded membrane structures with visual pigments.
- Inner segment contains the nucleus and organelles.
- Innermost structure is a synaptic terminal.

Fig. 7.7 compares the connections and functions of rods and cones.

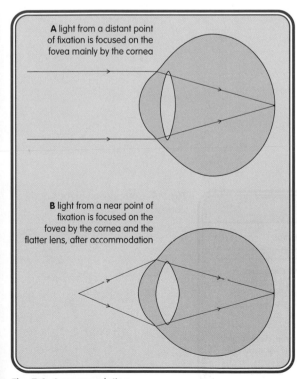

A light from a distant point of fixation is focused on the fovea mainly by the cornea

B light from a near point of fixation is focused on the fovea by the cornea and the flatter lens, after accommodation

Fig. 7.3 Accommodation.

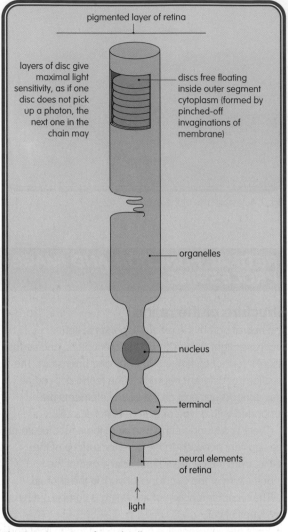

pigmented layer of retina

layers of disc give maximal light sensitivity, as if one disc does not pick up a photon, the next one in the chain may

discs free floating inside outer segment cytoplasm (formed by pinched-off invaginations of membrane)

organelles

nucleus

terminal

neural elements of retina

light

Fig. 7.5 Structure of a rod cell.

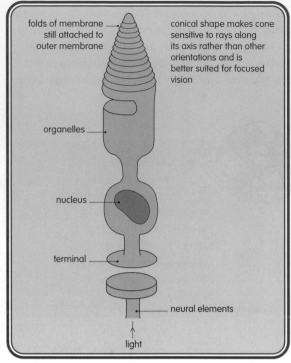

folds of membrane still attached to outer membrane

conical shape makes cone sensitive to rays along its axis rather than other orientations and is better suited for focused vision

organelles

nucleus

terminal

neural elements

light

Fig. 7.6 Structure of a cone cell.

Fig. 7.7 Comparison of rods and cones.

Comparison of rods and cones				
Receptor	Total number	Location	Connection to output cells	Function
Rod	120×10^6	peripheral retina, around the fovea	convergent pattern where many rods send information to a few output cells and this compresses information	responding to dim light with low spatial resolution and mediating visual reflexes from stimuli in the peripheral field
Cone	6×10^6	clustered in the fovea	no convergence; each cone projects to one bipolar cell, which projects to one output cell	focused, highly detailed colour vision with high spatial resolution

Visual pigments

Visual pigments undergo chemical change as a result of absorbing the energy from photons, enabling transduction of light into a neural signal. The pigments used by the rod system and the cone system differ, reflecting their different functions.

Visual pigments have a characteristic structure consisting of the vitamin A aldehyde, retinal, covalently attached to a protein, one of the opsins. The second-messenger system that the opsins modulate involves cyclic guanosine monophosphate, cGMP (opsins resemble G-protein-coupled receptors).

In rods, the pigment is rhodopsin. Its protein component, called opsin, lies in the membrane of the intracytoplasmic discs in the rod, with seven membrane-spanning domains (Fig. 7.8) arranged around the retinal molecule, which attaches to the seventh transmembrane domain.

In cones, the variation in pigment is produced by different forms of opsin with their own specific interaction with 11-*cis*-retinal. This results in the different absorption sensitivities in the cone system:

- B cones at 420 nm (blue).
- G cones at 531 nm (green).
- R cones at 558 nm (red).

The activation cascade for signalling that light has reached the rod or cone outer segment, shown in Fig. 7.9, begins with the change in retinal and ends with an alteration in membrane permeability to cations.

The photosensitive part of rhodopsin is retinal, which in the inactivated state is in the 11-*cis* configuration; after light absorption there is a rotation about the 11-*cis* double bond, producing the all-*trans* configuration. This disrupts the binding of retinal to opsin and the two separate, producing a conformational change in opsin.

Opsin reduces cGMP levels by a G-protein transducin and the cGMP hydrolyser, cGMP phosphodiesterase.

In darkness the cGMP-gated channels in the outer segment membrane are open because there has been no photon-instigated reduction in the intracellular level of cGMP. The steady inflow of Na^+ (the 'dark current') keeps the resting membrane of the receptor at −40 mV, producing a constant release of the neurotransmitter glutamate at its synapse.

After a reduction in cGMP the channels close, hyperpolarizing the cell and reducing glutamate release at the synapse. Greater light intensities produce greater

hyperpolarization (up to a maximum of −70 mV with all the Na^+ channels closed).

The pigment epithelium recycles the all-*trans* retinal, converting it back to the 11-*cis* form and transporting it back to the photoreceptors with a binding protein. It also phagocytoses the membrane of the photoreceptors to allow regrowth, as radiation destroys the membrane. Rods are phagocytosed during the day and cones at night.

Connections in the retina

Fig. 7.10 shows the circuit in the retina. There are excitatory and inhibitory connections between photoreceptors and bipolar cells, depending on the postsynaptic glutamate receptor on the bipolar cell. Remember that light stimulation reduces glutamate release.

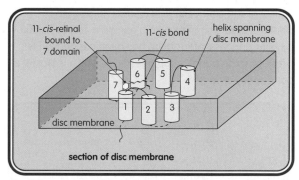

Fig. 7.8 Structure of rhodopsin, showing the seven-helix structure similar to the G-protein coupled receptor.

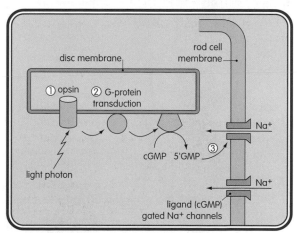

Fig. 7.9 Signal transduction of light impulses.
(1) Conformational change. Afterwards, all-*trans* retinal no longer binds, which affects the G-protein transduction.
(2) Increased activity of cGMP phosphodiesterase, which hydrolyses cGMP, reducing its intracellular level.
(3) Low cGMP levels close the ligand-gated channels, and thereby hyperpolarize the rod.

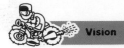

- For inhibitory (hyperpolarizing) synapses, reduction in glutamate release in response to illumination produces depolarization of the bipolar cell.
- For excitatory (depolarizing) synapses, reduction in glutamate release will hyperpolarize the bipolar cell.

All bipolar cells excite ganglion cells.

The receptive field of a ganglion cell is the region of retina which, when stimulated, affects the firing of the ganglion cell. The size and properties of the receptive field of the ganglion cell are determined by the number of photoreceptors it is connected to via the bipolar cells and the type of connections between the photoreceptors and bipolar cells.

If many receptors converge on a ganglion cell via bipolar cells, its receptive field will be very large, condensing a lot of information into one signal, which is typical of rod connections. If a small number of photoreceptors converge on a ganglion cell, its field is smaller and less information has been condensed in producing the ganglion output signal, which is typical of cone connections.

The characteristic ganglion-cell receptive field is circular, with either an excitatory or inhibitory response from a central zone and the opposite response in the surrounding peripheral zone.

Direct receptor–bipolar–ganglion connections produce responses in the central field and connections through horizontal interneurons produce the opposite responses in the peripheral field. These fields are described as having an on-centre/off-surround or off-centre/on-surround, as shown in Fig. 7.11.

Ganglion cell activity will be greatest when there is a contrast between the centre and the surround. If the whole field is illuminated or in darkness there is minimal activity because the two antagonistic responses cancel each other out. This response pattern helps the visual system to respond to contrast in the visual scene.

There are two major types of ganglion cell—one responding to change in the visual scene and the other to detail. A third type is likely to be involved in visual reflexes and eye movements. Their properties are summarized in Fig. 7.12.

Fig. 7.10 Processing of visual information in the retinal layers. (ONL, outer nuclear layer; OPL, outer plexiform layer; INL, inner nuclear layer; IPL, inner plexiform layer; GCL, ganglion cell layer.)

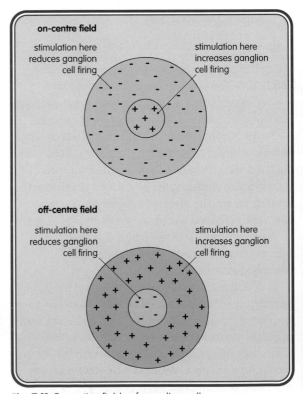

Fig. 7.11 Receptive fields of ganglion cells.

Fig. 7.12 Retinal ganglion cell types.

Ganglion cell	Structure	Receptive field	Response properties	Projection site	Function
Retinal ganglion cell types					
X	small cell, small dendritic arbor	small	wavelength specific, slowly adapting	thalamus	signals fine detail and colour
Y	large cell, large dendritic arbor	large	rapidly adapting	thalamus, midbrain	signals movement and illumination
W	large cell, large dendritic arbor	large	variable	midbrain	involved in eye movement control

Horizontal integration

Boundaries between light and dark (i.e. edges of objects) are enhanced by the horizontal connections provided by cells in the plexiform layers. The horizontal cells in the outer plexiform layer contact a number of photoreceptors and bipolar cells and as a result can integrate information from illuminated and non-illuminated areas of the retina.

- **Which biochemical processes convert the energy of photons into modulations in a second-messenger pathway?**
- **Discuss the visual pigments in colour vision.**
- **Describe the structure of rods and cones.**
- **Summarize the circuit of cells in the retina and their functions.**
- **How do retinal circuits produce the receptive field of the ganglion cells?**
- **What is the significance of the ganglion cell receptive field and the different response properties of ganglion cells?**

CENTRAL VISUAL PATHWAYS AND THE VISUAL CORTEX

Central visual pathways

The major projection from the ganglion cells passes in the optic nerve to the lateral geniculate nucleus of the thalamus, where the axons synapse on cells projecting to the visual cortex.

A smaller projection synapses in the midbrain (pretectal area and superior colliculus), controlling visual reflexes and eye movements; there is a small projection from here to higher visual processing areas.

The hemispheres process visual information from only one side of the visual axis (the contralateral), but the optic nerve leaving each eye contains information from both sides of the axis. Some fibres therefore need to cross over so that they project to the contralateral thalamus and this occurs at the chiasm in front of the pituitary stalk, as shown in Fig. 7.13.

The effects of lesions of the central pathway on visual function are dependent on the site of damage. These are summarized in Fig. 12.11.

Thalamus and visual cortex
The lateral geniculate nucleus

The optic nerve termination in the lateral geniculate nucleus is separated by eye (thus lateral geniculate nucleus cells receive monocular information) and by ganglion cell type.

The retinal fibres terminate in six discrete layers—four parvocellular layers and two magnocellular layers. Each eye transmits to three of the layers with the small-field X-ganglion cells projecting to two parvocellular

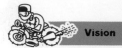
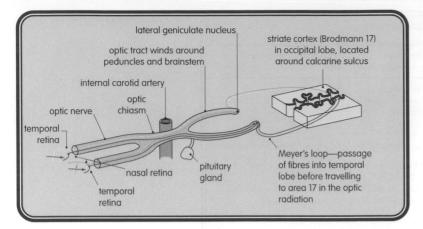

Fig. 7.13 Central visual pathway.

Figure labels:
- lateral geniculate nucleus
- optic tract winds around peduncles and brainstem
- internal carotid artery
- optic chiasm
- optic nerve
- temporal retina
- nasal retina
- temporal retina
- pituitary gland
- striate cortex (Brodmann 17) in occipital lobe, located around calcarine sulcus
- Meyer's loop—passage of fibres into temporal lobe before travelling to area 17 in the optic radiation

layers (whose cells are concerned with fine detail), and the large-field Y-cells to one magnocellular layer (whose cells are concerned with movement).

The lateral geniculate nucleus has a retinotopic organization, meaning that a given area of the retina will project to only a certain part of the lateral geniculate nucleus. Cells that receive inputs from the same area of the retina are stacked in columns running perpendicular to the layers.

Cells in the lateral geniculate nucleus have the same response properties as retinal ganglion cells—small circular fields with centre/surround interactions.

There are non-retinal inputs to the lateral geniculate nucleus (from the visual cortex and the pontine reticular formation) that can alter the traffic of information to the visual cortex. This can accentuate information of special interest, which is a mechanism of attention.

The visual cortex

The visual cortex lies along the calcarine sulcus on the medial aspect of the occipital lobe. The lateral geniculate nucleus projects a distorted retinotopic map onto the primary visual area (V1), Brodmann's area 17, so that information from the fovea gains access to a larger volume of cortex than information from the peripheral retina, as shown in Fig. 7.14.

Cells in the magnocellular and parvocellular layers in the lateral geniculate nucleus terminate in layer 4 of the V1 cortex. Other lateral geniculate nucleus cells (interlaminar cells) terminate in layers 2 and 3 on patches of cells termed 'blobs' (see below).

Response of V1 neurons and functional arrangement

Most V1 neurons respond to lines or edges (orientation selectivity), unlike retinal and lateral geniculate nucleus neurons, which have circular receptive fields. Cells that respond to similar line orientations are collected in columns perpendicular to the cortical surface (orientation columns).

Orientation-selective cells can be further classified:

- Simple cells respond to light/dark edges at a specific orientation in a restricted part of the visual field—imagine that they add up the input from adjacent ganglion cells so that the line is a series of small circles.

- Complex cells respond similarly but in a much larger area of the visual field, and maximally to the movement of the edge across the receptive field—imagine that they add up the input from simple cells.

For both cell types, moving stimuli produce better responses than static ones and certain directions of movement produce better responses than others.

The orientation columns are grouped together into units that are capable of responding to all orientations of lines in the same part of the visual field. These units are called hypercolumns, as shown in Fig. 7.15.

Within the hypercolumn the orientation columns are arranged so that the inputs from the left and right eyes are kept separate, forming so-called ocular dominance columns. This enables higher processing areas to compare the information from both eyes to create depth perception.

Within the hypercolumns there are regions between groups of orientation columns, called 'blob' regions. These are made up of groups of cells responding to colour contrast, with the centre/surround interaction response pattern to a primary colour (centre) and its complement (surround).

Progression of visual processing

The visual scene that we 'see' is built up from different processing circuits in the visual cortex. The processing circuits are formed by pathways through separate areas of the visual cortex each of which contain a retinotopic map. This allows representation of different types of activity in the visual field.

There are three pathways processing colour, motion and form. Things are not as simple as that because of the interconnections between the pathways but the major differences between them are summarized in Fig. 7.16.

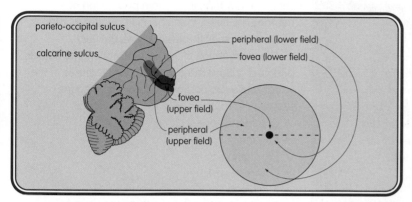

Fig. 7.14 Primary visual cortex—location and representation.

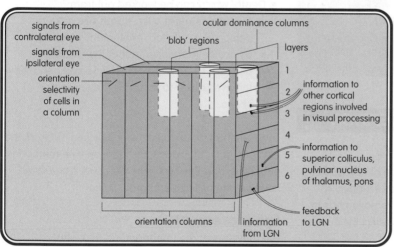

Fig. 7.15 A hypercolumn processing colour and line information from one part of the visual field. (LGN, lateral geniculate nucleus.)

Fig. 7.16 The three visual pathways.

The three visual pathways				
Basic function	Ganglion cell	Visual cortical regions in pathway	Responses of cells	Perceptual role
Motion	Y	V1, V2, V3, V5, then to parietal lobe	rapid responses for moving stimuli, no sensitivity to colour	detection of motion and arrangement of objects
Form	X	V1, V2, V4, then to parietal lobe and temporal lobe	slowing adapting, some colour sensitivity sensitive to orientation of edges	detection of shape of stationary objects
Colour	X	V1, V2, V4, then to temporal lobe	colour sensitive	detection of colour

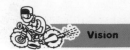

○ **What is the anatomical position and structure of the central visual pathway? How can it be affected by disease of closely related structures?**

○ **Summarize the arrangement of the lateral geniculate nucleus.**

○ **How is the visual cortex arranged into different areas? Discuss the functional organization of area V1.**

○ **What changes occur in the response properties of neurons during visual processing?**

○ **How is the visual image created? Describe the basic function and response properties of cells in the three processing pathways.**

ATTENTION AND PERCEPTION

Attention

The process of attention is the selection of a focus from sensory information in order to process it further. A certain amount of processing of all information has to occur before attentional mechanisms select the appropriate information.

Attending to a part of our environment involves visual and motor mechanisms to orient the body in space, allowing us to scan the visual field or interact with the environment in motor tasks.

The factors that determine where attention is directed are novelty and relevance to current tasks.

Certain types of visual input are processed fully before any type of selection occurs. When we look at words we can not stop ourselves reading and understanding them—we never just see lines on a page after we have learned to read.

Perception

The process of perception involves representing the contents of the environment and then making sense of the representation (e.g. by organizing visual information into objects and background, and then identifying the objects).

Representation of the environment in the visual cortex is achieved by the retinotopic maps. Higher centres know that, if a certain population of V1 neurons are firing, then specific boundaries are present in a specific part of the visual field.

The segregation of visual information into objects and background relies upon certain features of the visual scene. Objects are picked out using the following list of principles:

- Common shape, colour, or texture.
- Continuity.
- Proximity.
- Common size.
- Closure.
- Depth, which can be worked out from:
  - monocular information about size, texture, perspective, overlap, movement parallax, or
  - binocular information about the difference between the view from the eyes and about how the eyes move to focus on the same part of space.

The identification of objects, once picked out from the environment, relies upon comparison with memories of objects, and this occurs in the visual association cortex at the occipitotemporal junction.

Eye movements

Eye movements are important in attentional mechanisms as they direct the fovea onto points of interest in the visual scene quickly and accurately. There are five types of eye movement, two of which stabilize the eye when the head moves:

- Vestibulo-ocular—uses vestibular input to hold the retinal image stable during brief or rapid head rotation. For horizontal movements, lateral rectus motor neurons (VI nucleus) are influenced by vestibular nuclei cells, medial rectus motor neurons (III nucleus) are driven by interneurons in the contralateral abducens nucleus.

- Optokinetic—uses visual input to hold the retinal image stable during sustained or slow head rotation. The underlying pathway comprises a retinal projection via the tectum to the vestibular nucleus and a cortical component from V1.

The other three eye movements keep the fovea on a visual target:
- Saccade—brings new objects of interest onto the fovea. They are very fast and occur every 300 ms. The pattern of saccadic eye movements is guided by current cognitive tasks, as shown by recordings of eye movements when pictures are scanned for details. Horizontal saccadic movements are generated in the pontine reticular formation, and vertical ones in the midbrain, under influence from a circuit involving the frontal eye fields (in the frontal lobes), the pulvinar nucleus of the thalamus, and the superior colliculus.
- Smooth pursuit—holds the image of a moving target on the fovea. This type of movement is controlled by visual and frontal cortical areas, relaying information to the vestibulocerebellum.
- Vergence—adjusts the eyes for differing image distances. This movement is controlled by midbrain neurons near the oculomotor nucleus

Smooth pursuit movements and saccadic eye movements can alternate (e.g. when looking out of a train window) and this combination of movements is termed optokinetic nystagmus.

Strategies in visual processing
There are two strategies employed by the visual system to make sense of the visual environment.
- Bottom-up processing occurs when a visual scene is analysed purely in terms of the incoming visual information, without searching visual memory for similar scenes that might help with making sense of the scene.
- Top-down processing occurs when visual memory influences the way in which the current visual scene is processed, so that some sort of sense can be made of the way in which objects are distinguished from their background.

Disorders of attention and perception
In the condition of neglect, patients fail to turn their attention to areas in the visual scene on one-half of space, typically the side of space contralateral to a parietal lobe lesion. They will entirely ignore one side of their visual axis, e.g. eating only half the food on a plate, or describing only half of a visual scene (when looking at it and when recollecting it).

In the condition of agnosia, patients cannot recognize objects from visual examination, although they can fully describe the physical features of the object (and recognize it from tactile information). Here there is a failure of the higher processes of perception that integrate all the visual information about an object and compare it with visual memory.

These conditions differ in important respects—in agnosia there is a failure of recognition of an object wherever it is in the visual field and in neglect there is a failure to attend to one-half of space, whatever objects lie therein.

- Describe 'attention' in terms of information processing.
- Discuss 'perception' in terms of the organization of visual input.
- Why are eye movements important for attention?
- Distinguish between bottom-up and top-down processing.
- Distinguish between disorders of attention and disorders of perception.

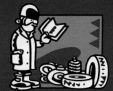

8. Hearing

THE EAR AND CONDUCTION OF SOUND

Sound waves are propagated variations in air pressure (i.e. alternating increased and decreased pressure) and propagated disturbances of the particles in the medium conducting the sound. The intensity of a sound wave is equal to the product of the pressure increase (or decrease) and the volume velocity (average particle velocity × area of the conducting medium).

There is a vast range of sound intensities detectable by the normal human auditory system (the loudest is 10^{12} times the auditory threshold); therefore, sound intensity is measured using a logarithmic scale with the unit of the decibel (dB).

The auditory system consists of the hearing apparatus (outer ear, middle ear, and inner ear) and a pathway from the inner ear to the brainstem and auditory cortex.

Anatomy of the auditory apparatus

Fig. 8.1 depicts the auditory apparatus.

Outer ear

The pinna and external ear canal form a tube closed at one end by the tympanic membrane and this tube has a resonant frequency of 3 kHz. This decreases the threshold for hearing by 15 dB in the frequency range 2.5–4 kHz.

Middle ear

Alternating air pressure (the sound wave) makes the tympanic membrane vibrate. This vibration is carried down the chain of ossicles to the base plate of the stapes in the oval window. The surface area of the base plate is much less than that of the tympanic membrane, amplifying the pressure changes. This minimizes the attenuation normally caused when sound waves travel from a less dense medium (air) to a more dense one (water).

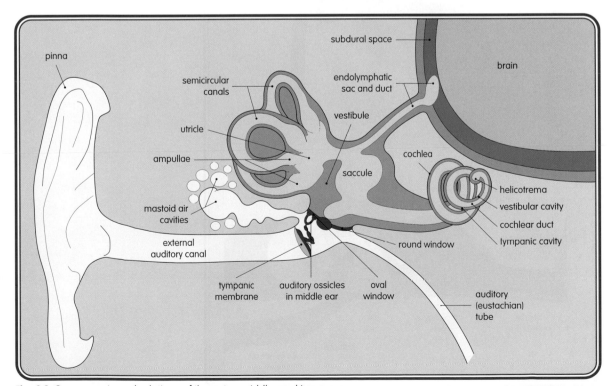

Fig. 8.1 Components and relations of the outer, middle, and inner ear.

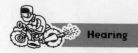

Vibrations of the ossicular chain are dampened down when they become extreme by the action of tensor tympani muscle on the malleus and the action of stapedius muscle on the stapes.

Inner ear

The cochlea is a spiral tunnel divided into three compartments running the length of the cochlea. The upper compartment (scala vestibuli) and lower compartment (scala tympani) communicate at the apex of the spiral (at the helicotrema) and contain a fluid called perilymph resembling cerebrospinal fluid. The base plate vibration causes movement in the perilymph in the scala vestibuli.

The cochlear duct lies between the scala vestibuli and the scala tympani, and contains a fluid called endolymph that has a high potassium concentration and a high positive potential with respect to the perilymph. The organ of Corti rests on the basilar membrane inside the cochlear duct, as shown in

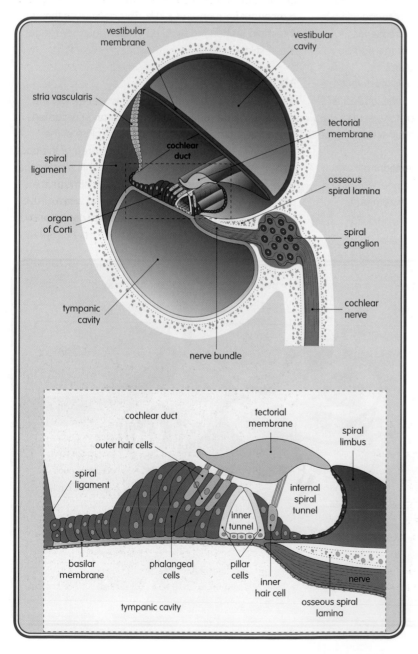

Fig. 8.2 The organ of Corti, lying in the cochlea.

Fig. 8.2, and perilymph movement makes the basilar membrane vibrate.

This vibrational movement is transmitted to the hair cells in the organ of Corti, which convert vibrations of their cilia into oscillating changes in their membrane potential. Cranial nerve VIII afferent neurons, whose cell bodies lie in the bony spiral lamina, contact the hair cells and send auditory information to the cochlear nuclei in the brainstem.

The organ of Corti

The ability to detect different frequencies of sound is given by properties of the basilar membrane and hair cells.

The basilar membrane increases in width as it winds round the cochleas so that its transverse fibres are longer at the top than at the bottom. Longer fibres have a lower resonant frequency and shorter ones have a higher resonant frequency.

The stiffness of the basilar membrane decreases 100-fold from base to apex. The electrical and mechanical properties of the hair cells vary along the basilar membrane. There is a reduction in the frequency of membrane potential resonance and a reduction in stiffness of stereocilia from the base to apex. Therefore, afferent fibres from the apical part of the cochlea carry low-frequency sound signals and afferent fibres from the basal part of the cochlea carry high-frequency sound signals.

Pure tones will cause most of the basilar membrane to vibrate, but they can be perceived because a narrow region of fibres will have a greater amplitude of vibration than the rest of the fibres.

Transduction of vibration

The hair cells convert oscillating movements of stereocilia into neuronal signals.

Vibrations of the basilar membrane result in oscillating movement of the hair cells. The stereocilia projecting from the upper surface of the hair cells are fixed at the extracellular end to the immobile tectorial membrane and sway with the same frequency as the part of the basilar membrane that the hair cells rest upon.

This results in oscillating changes in the physical arrangement of the hair cell membrane and,

consequently, oscillating changes in the structure of membrane ion channels. Fluctuations in ion permeability are produced, which result in oscillations of membrane potential with the same frequency as the basilar membrane.

Control over sensitivity

Hair cells are arranged in rows on either side of the pillar cells—three rows of outer cells and one row of inner cells. The inner and outer rows have different functions based on the different proportions of output-signalling fibres and input-controlling fibres that contact them.

More afferent neurons contact the base of the inner cells (they signal sound) and more efferents contact the base of the outer cells (they stiffen their cilia in response and lift the tectorial membrane upwards, decreasing the response of the inner cells to basilar membrane vibration).

Tonotopic mapping

The spatial separation of frequencies in the cochlea leads to frequency selectivity of the cells to which cochlear nerve fibres project. This means that there is a frequency map in the auditory cortex. Cochlea implants use this spatial selectivity of response.

Sound can be conducted through bone. Thus, after middle ear damage, some hearing may be preserved by relying on bone conduction.

- **How do the structures of the external ear, middle ear ossicles, cochlea, and basilar membrane produce selective responses in the auditory system?**
- **Explain the process of auditory signal transduction.**
- **Contrast the functions of the inner and outer hair cells.**

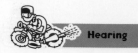

THE CENTRAL AUDITORY PATHWAYS AND THE AUDITORY CORTEX

Central auditory pathways

The pathways are organized so that:

- The differential frequency selectivity given by the cochlea is retained throughout the pathways by an orderly projection of frequencies (tonotopic projection) to different areas of the primary auditory cortex.
- Inputs from both ears interact with each other in the process of sound localization.

Fig. 8.3 shows that cochlear nerve afferent fibres terminate in the dorsal and ventral cochlear nuclei, preserving their tonotopic organization. From here there are two main pathways:

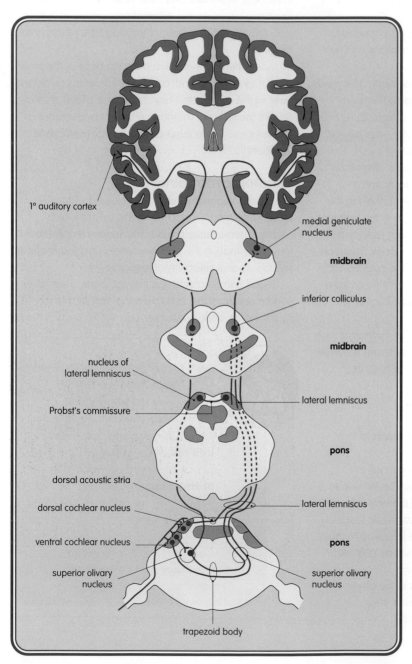

Fig. 8.3 Central auditory pathways.

1° auditory cortex

medial geniculate nucleus

midbrain

inferior colliculus

midbrain

nucleus of lateral lemniscus

lateral lemniscus

Probst's commissure

pons

dorsal acoustic stria

lateral lemniscus

dorsal cochlear nucleus

ventral cochlear nucleus

pons

superior olivary nucleus

superior olivary nucleus

trapezoid body

- The dorsal acoustic stria.
- The trapezoid body, which carries fibres to the superior olivary nucleus on both sides of the pons.

The superior olive is a contact point between the left and right cochlear nuclei and allows comparison between sound input for localization.

Fibres from the superior olive project to the inferior colliculus in the lateral lemniscus, with fibres from the cochlear nuclei. Some are interrupted, synapsing in the nucleus of the lateral lemniscus where there is further communication with the contralateral auditory input through Probst's commissure.

Fibres from the inferior colliculus project to the medial geniculate nucleus of the thalamus and from there to the primary auditory cortex, on the superomedial aspect of the temporal lobe.

Damage to one side of the auditory pathway at any level (other than the cochlear nerve) will not result in deafness in one ear. This is because of the bilateral projections to the auditory cortex, both directly and by communication between pathways.

Auditory cortex

The auditory cortex is functionally organized into maps of the frequency range that we can hear (so-called tonotopic organization).

Cells responding to input from both ears to varying degrees are arranged into columns. Within a column the cells have the same binaural response properties. There are two types of column, which alternate across the cortex:

- Suppression columns, where cells respond more strongly to input from one ear and these may be involved in sound localization.
- Summation columns, where cells respond more strongly to input from both ears.

The cortex uses differences in sound intensity and time of arrival at the ear to localize sounds, and the function of each hemisphere is to localize sound from the contralateral side of space. From 200 Hz to 2000 Hz, the process involves interaural delay; from 2000 Hz to 20 000 Hz, it involves interaural intensity differences.

Speech processing

In most people, one hemisphere carries out language processing and is called the dominant hemisphere, usually being the left hemisphere for both right-handed and left-handed people.

Wernicke's area in the temporal lobe on the dominant side is an auditory association area that integrates sound information so that meaningful speech can be recognized. It codes sounds into phonemes, which are the most basic sound units of spoken language.

Broca's area in the frontal lobe on the dominant side processes the motor programmes that are sent to the vocal muscles, producing speech. It matches up a desired phoneme with the motor commands to produce that phoneme.

In speech production, connections between Wernicke's area and Broca's area ensure that the sounds that we wish to make are actually made.

Speech processing involves other areas, such as the frontal lobe (Fig. 8.4).

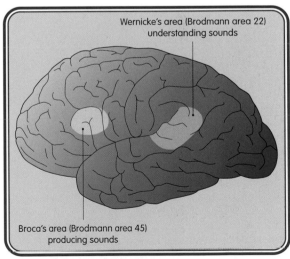

Fig. 8.4 Location of Broca's and Wernicke's areas in the dominant hemisphere.

- What are the bilateral projections to the auditory cortex? Explain the function of this arrangement.
- Describe the tonotopic organization of the auditory cortex and the binaural response properties of its cells.
- Summarize the anatomical basis of speech processing.

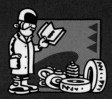

9. Olfaction and Taste

RECEPTORS FOR TASTE AND SMELL

Taste receptors

Clusters (50–150) of taste receptors are found in the 2000–5000 taste buds in the epithelial layer of the tongue, palate, and pharynx. The base of each receptor cell is innervated by a branch of a primary afferent fibre, forming a synaptic structure. In the tongue, taste buds are located on different types of papillae, as shown in Fig. 9.1.

Signal transduction varies for the four taste modalities:

- Saltiness is detected by Na^+ ions passing through an amiloride-sensitive channel to depolarize the receptor cell membrane, resulting in transmitter release that activates the primary afferent fibre.
- Sourness is caused by H^+-ion production by acids. These depolarize the cell in two ways: directly by passing through amiloride-sensitive Na^+ channels, causing an inward current, and indirectly by binding to and blocking K^+ channels, which also causes depolarization.
- Sweetness is signalled when molecules bind to a specific receptor site coupled to a G-protein. This triggers an increase in cytoplasmic cAMP, which then activates protein kinase A; this, in turn, phosphorylates K^+ channels, which become blocked. This leads to depolarization.
- Bitterness receptors are essentially poison detectors. Some bitter compounds (e.g. quinine) bind directly to and block K^+ channels. Other compounds bind to specific bitter membrane receptors that activate G-protein second-messenger cascades. One type of bitter receptor produces an increase in intracellular inositol triphosphate, causing intracellular Ca^{2+} release, which leads to transmitter release and afferent nerve activation.

Most taste receptor cells respond to two or more of the basic tastes. Tastes are not synthesized from stimulation of four distinct pathways. Taste afferent neurons are less specific than the receptors because one afferent can innervate several papillae, and in the solitary nucleus a single cell can receive synapses from many taste afferent neurons. Taste has to be interpreted from broadly tuned input channels.

The brain may interpret taste using other inputs such as smell, temperature, and texture.

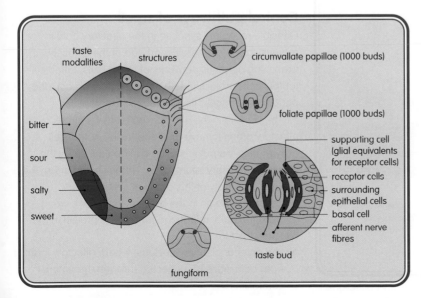

Fig. 9.1 Structure of a taste bud and location of different papillae and taste modalities on the tongue.

Olfactory receptors

Olfactory receptors are located in the epithelial lining of the nasal cavity, as shown in Fig. 9.2, in an area known as the olfactory epithelium.

Mechanisms of the sense of smell

Odour enter the mucus film of the olfactory epithelium and diffuse to the receptor cell cilia. Interaction with specific binding proteins on the ciliary surface results in changes in a second-messenger pathway, possibly involving cAMP, opening Na^+ channels and producing depolarization in the region of the cilia.

There are many olfactory receptor proteins, which allow recognition of thousands of different odorants and at very low concentrations (parts per 10^{12}).

○ **Describe the principles of signal transduction for olfactory and gustatory stimuli. Where are the receptors located?**
○ **Relate the response properties of the receptor systems to the human capabilities of taste and smell.**

CENTRAL PATHWAYS OF TASTE AND SMELL

Central pathways of taste

The taste pathway does not cross over the midline and so the hemispheres process ipsilateral gustatory stimuli.

Taste receptors synapse on afferent neurons of cranial nerve VII, IX, or X, depending on their location. The afferent neurons pass into the medulla where they synapse in a part of the solitary nucleus called the gustatory nucleus.

The gustatory nucleus projects to the thalamus (ventroposterior medial nucleus) and from the thalamus there are projections to the sensory cortex and the insula (Fig. 9.3).

Central pathways of smell

Olfactory receptors synapse in the olfactory bulb in regions called 'glomeruli' made up of the diffusely branching dendritic networks of mitral cells, tufted cells (output cells projecting to higher olfactory areas), and periglomerular cells (local inhibitory neurons).

The circuitry in the olfactory bulb allows higher olfactory areas to have an influence on output cell activity; also, output inhibition can be caused by the incoming olfactory information. This is shown in Fig. 9.4.

The complexity of this circuit allows olfactory processing to begin in the bulb.

From the bulb, mitral and tufted cells project in the olfactory tract to:
• The anterior olfactory nucleus, where olfactory input from both sides is connected through the anterior commissure.

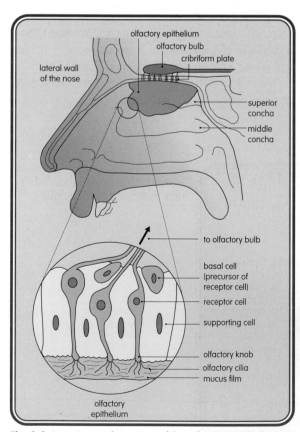

Fig. 9.2 Location and structure of the olfactory epithelium.

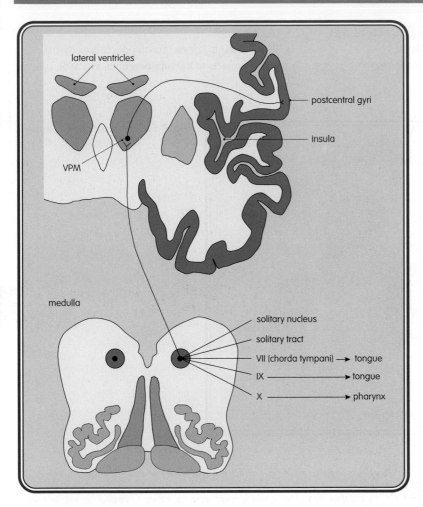

Fig. 9.3 Central pathway of taste. (VPM, ventral posterior medial nucleus.)

lateral ventricles

postcentral gyri

Insula

VPM

medulla

solitary nucleus

solitary tract

VII (chorda tympani) → tongue

IX → tongue

X → pharynx

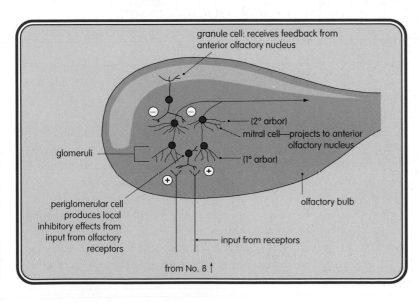

Fig. 9.4 Influences on the efferent fibres from the olfactory bulb.

granule cell: receives feedback from anterior olfactory nucleus

(2° arbor)

mitral cell—projects to anterior olfactory nucleus

glomeruli

(1° arbor)

periglomerular cell produces local inhibitory effects from input from olfactory receptors

input from receptors

olfactory bulb

from No. 8 ↑

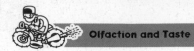

- The olfactory tubercle, which has connections with the thalamus (medial dorsal nucleus).
- The pyriform cortex, which processes the discrimination between odours.

- The amygdala.
- The entorhinal cortex (parahippocampal gyrus), which projects to the hippocampus (Fig. 9.5).

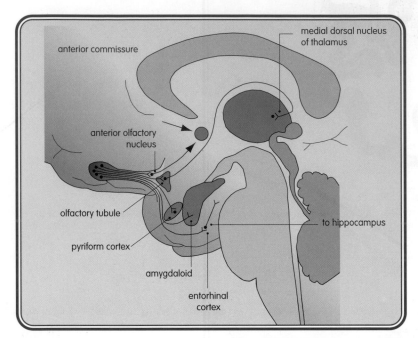

Fig. 9.5 Central pathway of smell.

⦿ **Describe the taste pathway through the medulla to the cortex.**
⦿ **Describe the circuitry in the olfactory bulb and the pathway to the different parts of the olfactory cortex.**

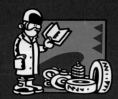

10. Higher Centres of the Central Nervous System

LOCALIZATION OF BRAIN FUNCTION AND BEHAVIOUR

Structural and functional asymmetry

There are structural differences between hemispheres. The planum temporale (superior aspect of the temporal lobe lying within the lateral sulcus) is larger on the left side. Wernicke's area lies in the posterior part of the planum temporale and this is often used as evidence that the brain has a preprogrammed language area on the left side.

Although the left and right hemispheres are connected through the corpus callosum, they carry out different functions. The evidence for this comes from:

- Patients with lesions localized to one hemisphere.
- Patients with severe grand mal epilepsy who have undergone sectioning of the corpus callosum (commissurotomy) to prevent spread of seizures.
- Normal subjects who are presented lateralized tasks so that only one hemisphere can process the stimuli.
- Positron emission tomography (PET) or functional magnetic resonance imaging (fMRI) of normal subjects performing a range of tasks.
- Wada's test, where amylobarbitone sodium is injected into one carotid artery, which temporarily anaesthetizes one hemisphere so that tasks can be processed only by the other one.

The left hemisphere processes information sequentially and so is involved in calculation and language (speech, writing, and verbally expressed thought).

The right hemisphere processes information by taking in the 'whole picture' and it performs 'gestalt' functions such as spatial construction and ideas that are not expressed verbally (depth judgements, spatial positioning).

It must be remembered that lateralization of function is not absolute. In the majority of right-handed and left-handed people the left hemisphere is dominant for language, but in a small proportion of both (larger for left-handers) both hemispheres share language processing more or less equally.

There is an element of plasticity in the location of function. In children who sustain damage to one hemisphere, the other one can take over the functions so that there is no appreciable deficit. This is not the case in adults, as shown by the effects of a cerebrovascular accident.

Cortical localization

Different cortical regions perform different functions. This is because of their different input and output connections.

Regions within different lobes can be split up into functional units:

- Primary sensory or motor areas, which receive information from outside the brain or project outside the brain.
- Higher-order sensory or motor areas, which are limited to processing sensory information from one modality (e.g. V2–V5) or motor information (e.g. the supplementary motor area).
- Association areas, where information from different modalities is brought together for processing that encompasses more than just vision, hearing, etc.

The functions of association areas are often worked out by examining the effect on behaviour when they are lesioned and by the patterns of metabolic activity from PET scans when normal subjects perform appropriate tasks.

The frontal lobes have:

- An association area that plans sequences of responses, changes response patterns to fit current demands, and controls emotional states.
- Higher-order motor processing areas that have motor control functions for eye movements (the frontal eye fields) and speech (Broca's area on the dominant side).

Therefore frontal cortex damage can produce:

- Inability to organize responses to solve problems.
- An error pattern of perseveration in tasks where changing rules govern responses. The Wisconsin card-sorting test is based on asking a subject to sort cards according to one rule (e.g. same colour), and then the examiner changes the rule (e.g. to same pattern). The subject works out the new rule by feedback from the examiner about correct or

incorrect card sorting. Perseveration occurs when subjects do not change from using a previously correct rule that has become incorrect.

- Personality changes occuring along emotional dimensions, typically becoming more impulsive, aggressive, and subject to rapid changes in emotional state.
- Disordered eye movement scanning of a visual scene.
- Damage to Broca's area produces problems in speech production with hesitant, limited speech (described as 'telegrammatic').

The temporal lobes have:
- Association areas that are involved in learning.
- Higher-order sensory areas involved in speech recognition (Wernicke's area) and visual object recognition.

The consequences of temporal damage are:
- Disorders in learning verbal information in left-sided lesions.
- Disorders in learning visuospatial information in right-sided lesions.
- Problems in understanding spoken and written language but no reduction in fluency of language production, resulting in meaningless or irrelevant speech.
- Object agnosia, where patients cannot recognize objects from visual information but can do so from other modalities, e.g. touch.

The parietal lobes have:
- A primary sensory area receiving somatosensory information.
- A higher-order sensory area.
- An association area where many sensory modalities converge to build up a picture of how the body is positioned in the environment (incorporating attentional mechanisms) and how the environment is structured.

Parietal damage can therefore produce:
- Lack of conscious sensation on one half of the body.
- Attentional deficits presenting as neglect (usually of the left half of space after a right-sided lesion).
- Inability to make voluntary eye movements after bilateral parietal damage (Balint syndrome).
- Constructional apraxia, which is an inability to organize movement in space as tested by attempting to copy a figure by drawing (seen with right-sided lesions).
- Disorders of spatial awareness tested by route finding (mainly seen with right-sided lesions).

With right-sided lesions, each hemisphere represents the contralateral half of space in the parietal cortex. However, there is an unequal amount of space represented in each hemisphere. The left hemisphere represents only the right side of space. The right hemisphere represents the left and some of the right side of space—therefore the right side of space is over-represented.

This means that lesions of the left parietal cortex will not badly affect processing of the right side of space because this is also being carried out to an extent in the right parietal cortex.

Right-sided lesions will produce effects on the processing of the left half of space because it is not carried out anywhere else.

- **State the differences between primary sensory and motor areas, higher sensory and motor areas, and association areas.**
- **What are the structural and functional differences between the hemispheres?**
- **Relate the deficits after localized damage in the frontal, temporal, and parietal lobes to the functions of these areas.**

LEARNING AND MEMORY

Learning is the acquisition of new information. Memory is the retention of learned information, and can be fractionated into two basic parts:

- Declarative memory for facts (semantic memory) and events (episodic memory). This is easy both to acquire and to lose.
- Procedural memory for skills/behaviour, which is hard to acquire and also hard to lose (even in profound loss of declarative memory).

Declarative memory can be split into three parts, as shown in Fig. 10.1:

- Sensory memory.
- Working memory.
- Long-term memory.

Sensory memory

Sensory memory is a store of all the sensory information that has just been processed. It is held in stores that are modality specific (e.g. visual stores, tactile stores) with a very high capacity, but that are limited in the time during which information can be held (fading after 0.5 s).

There is no conscious access to sensory memory. Its function is in selective attention, filtering the inputs that will be consciously processed by working memory.

Working memory

Working memory contains the information that we are processing 'right now' and we have conscious access to it. Inputs to working memory are from sensory memory or long-term memory.

Its span (maximum capacity) is typically 7 ± 2 units of information (number, word, etc.), and the total amount of information it can store is increased by altering the unit coding strategy so that each unit contains more information.

It functions as a push-down stack, so that new units of information displace the oldest units from the working memory store.

It has a visual store and a verbal store. Words are more likely to be coded by their acoustic properties than by semantic properties (what the words mean).

A central processor determines the type of coding system for verbal information to be used and the focus of attention from the sensory memory store.

Long-term memory

Long-term memory is a collection of different types of memory that are differentiated by the nature of the information stored. As a general principle of long-term memory properties, these stores show unlimited capacity, but limitations in the capacity of the retrieval mechanism.

Distinctions between long-term memory and working memory
Studies of amnesia

In Wernicke–Korsakoff syndrome, the amnesia affects memory for events in adult life (sparing childhood memories) but patients have a preserved working memory span.

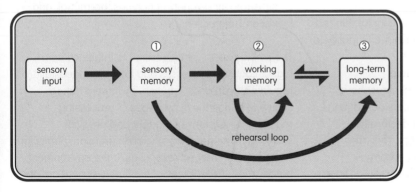

Fig. 10.1 The three-stage model of memory.

The serial position effect

After giving normal subjects a list of data, then asking them to recall the information freely in any order, the first units of information are recalled (the primacy effect) and the last units are recalled (the recency effect). After a delay before testing recall, the recency effect is lost. This suggests that working memory holds the most recently given data and that long-term memory is holding the first few units of information.

The coding strategy for holding verbal information

Working memory uses an acoustic strategy (evidence for this comes from error patterns made by normals when recalling verbal information) and long-term memory stores verbal information in terms of meaning (typically, we can remember the 'gist' of what people have said without recalling the actual words used).

Capacity for information

Working memory is limited in terms of the amount of information it holds and the time for which it is held. Long-term memory has an unlimited capacity for information and the information held has a much longer 'shelf life'.

Amnesia and localization of memory function

Amnesia is the loss of memory and/or the ability to learn, either caused by brain injury (organic amnesia) or for psychological reasons such as great stress (psychogenic amnesia).

Retrograde amnesia is a loss of memory for things before injury and anterograde amnesia is an inability to form new memories after injury.

Medial temporal lobe structures (e.g. hippocampus and parahippocampal gyrus) have been implicated in memory function, as damage in these areas produces disruption of declarative memory, sparing procedural memory. This area receives highly processed information from association cortices and, as a possible cellular basis for memory, the phenomenon of long-term potentiation (see below) has been recorded in cells in the hippocampus.

Memory disruption also occurs after frontal and thalamic lesions.

- State the distinctions between the types of memory and the functions of the three different parts of declarative memory.
- Summarize the evidence that indicates a distinction between working memory and long-term memory.
- Name the structures implicated in memory function.

THE LIMBIC SYSTEM

Overview of the limbic system

The limbic system is a complex system of fibre tracts and grey matter, located on the medial aspect of each hemisphere encircling (limbus = border) the upper part of the brainstem.

- It serves as the 'nervous system' for emotional feelings and behaviour.
- Its extensive connections to both lower and higher parts of the central nervous system give the system an ability to integrate a wide variety of stimuli.
- Its connections with the hypothalamus provide a substrate for a variety of nervous, hormonal, and visceral interactions.

The limbic system is in a position to influence both higher cognitive processes and lower homoeostatic regulatory processes. Emotion, by its very nature, seems to bridge these two types of processing, requiring dimensions of thought and physical sensations. Memory plays a role in emotion, particularly in guiding behavioural responses to the environment, but the memory functions of the limbic system are not restricted to emotionally laden stimuli.

Although this picture of different functions may seem confusing, it highlights the areas to be aware of when dealing with patients who have suffered damage to these regions.

Structure of the limbic system

Fig. 10.2 shows the arrangement of limbic structures. We can consider the complicated connections of the limbic system as two simpler systems:

- One primarily involved in learning and memory.
- One involved with the processing of emotion, particularly its behavioural and endocrine aspects.

There are modulatory inputs from the reticular formation. The locus ceruleus sends a noradrenergic input and the raphe nuclei send a serotoninergic input.

Hippocampal circuit

The hippocampal circuit runs from the medial temporal lobe (hippocampus and parahippocampal gyrus) to the mammillary bodies and thalamus, and is involved in learning and memory. The connections offer some guide as to how information flows in the circuit, as shown in Fig. 10.3.

There is some debate about the precise role of this circuit, particularly the hippocampus, parahippocampal gyrus, and mammillary bodies, but the following points are clear:

- Damage to the medial temporal lobe involving the hippocampus and parahippocampal gyrus (e.g. after herpes simplex encephalitis) produces a profound memory deficit.
- The physiological properties of cells in the hippocampus allow them to give increased responses to certain patterns of input. This occurs via long-term potentiation, which is an increase in the efficacy of a synapse, and would obviously have a role in keeping certain patterns of activity going. This could be one strategy in the neural basis of memory.
- Degeneration of the mammillary bodies occurs in Wernicke–Korsakoff syndrome, where a combination of alcohol abuse and thiamine deficiency results in a memory disorder with poor learning ability (anterograde amnesia) and poor recall of events before the onset of the disease (retrograde amnesia).

Amygdaloid circuit

This circuit is less clear in function, possibly as a result of its rather diffuse connections.

The amygdala is a collection of cell groups lying at the anterior tip of the medial temporal lobe just in front of the hippocampus. It can be divided up in terms of its connections, and also function, into two parts—one medial and one lateral.

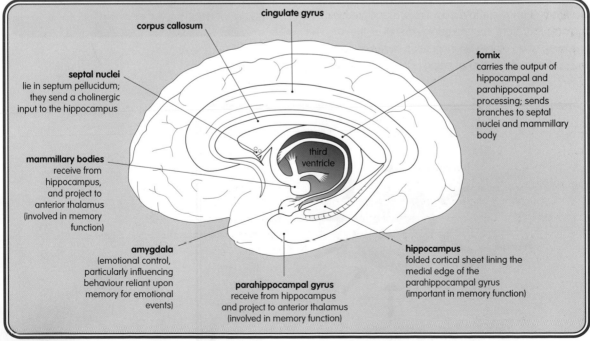

Fig. 10.2 Outline of the limbic system.

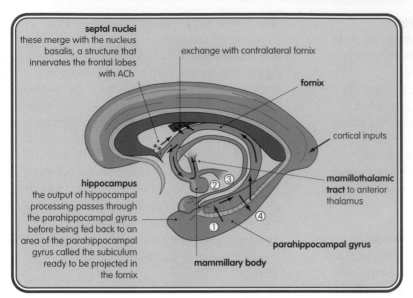

septal nuclei
these merge with the nucleus basalis, a structure that innervates the frontal lobes with ACh

exchange with contralateral fornix

fornix

cortical inputs

mamillothalamic tract to anterior thalamus

hippocampus
the output of hippocampal processing passes through the parahippocampal gyrus before being fed back to an area of the parahippocampal gyrus called the subiculum ready to be projected in the fornix

parahippocampal gyrus

mammillary body

Fig. 10.3 Processing in the hippocampal circuit. Direction of flow of processing is indicated by numbered arrows.

Fig. 10.4 shows inputs to the amygdala. Its outputs are simply connections travelling to the sources of input (reciprocal connections), but the largest output is to the hypothalamus through the stria terminalis.

There is potential for this circuit to carry out a number of different functions and there is little point in searching for a unifying theory that functionally links all the connections together. Lesion experiments on animals examining the function of the lateral part of the amygdala suggest that this circuit is involved in governing behaviour towards stimuli associated with reward. Therefore the amygdala can tell us the meaning of an otherwise innocuous stimulus, such as the perfume of a lover not being just another smell.

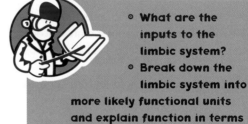

○ **What are the inputs to the limbic system?**
○ **Break down the limbic system into more likely functional units and explain function in terms of circuitry.**
○ **Describe the effects of damage in the limbic system.**

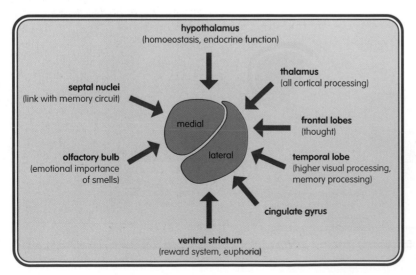

hypothalamus
(homoeostasis, endocrine function)

thalamus
(all cortical processing)

septal nuclei
(link with memory circuit)

medial

frontal lobes
(thought)

lateral

olfactory bulb
(emotional importance of smells)

temporal lobe
(higher visual processing, memory processing)

cingulate gyrus

ventral striatum
(reward system, euphoria)

Fig. 10.4 Connections of amygdala.

COGNITIVE DEVELOPMENT AND DEGENERATION

Cognitive development

Development is an alteration in function or ability. Cognitive development can be assessed either with set tasks such as learning tests or by observation of uninfluenced behaviour. It is therefore staged in terms of the emergence of certain behaviours or the ages at which certain tasks are achieved.

Many factors influence the rate of cognitive development and how far we will ultimately reach along a natural developmental axis. The chemical environment is crucial both *in utero* and in early childhood, as is nutritional status during this period. Depending on how one assesses cognitive function, the amount and quality of education will influence final performance.

An outline of development starts with the baseline abilities of newborn babies and then charts alterations in, or additions to, these abilities throughout childhood.

Ability of the newborn

The newborn's learning capabilities include:

- Auditory discrimination as well as localization of the sound source, tested by observing head movements.
- Operant learning where, if certain responses are rewarded, babies will be more likely to make those responses.

The newborn's perceptual capabilities:

- Are responses requiring coordination between sensory modalities, e.g. making eye movements towards a sound source.
- Include smooth pursuit eye movements.
- Respond preferentially (with more interest) to certain stimuli (e.g. human faces).

The newborn's motor capabilities are basic motor programmes (e.g. reaching movements if body weight is supported).

The social behaviour of the newborn is to interact with the primary care-giver by imitation of facial movements.

Motor changes

New motor abilities emerge in a set pattern, with the rate of appearance varying according to stimulation and in certain conditions (e.g. Down syndrome).

Visual input is crucial to the natural development of reaching movements. Babies who are congenitally blind need special devices, such as echo locators, to develop appropriate reaching movements.

The fundamental changes in motor development are greater control over fine movements and greater fluidity of a series of movements.

Perceptual changes

Changes in perceptual ability involve learning how to interpret sensory information. One milestone is the development of depth perception tested by Gibson's visual cliff experiment. An infant is allowed freely to explore a horizontal plane, part of which is transparent revealing a drop to floor level. During the period of crawling, infants will not cross the visual cliff onto the transparent area.

The rate of acquisition of knowledge about the environment limits the development of perceptual abilities and will also affect attentional mechanisms.

Overall scheme of cognitive development—Piaget's theory

Sensorimotor stage, 0–2 years

This stage is characterized by the development of object permanence, where infants understand that objects still exist when they can no longer perceive them (e.g. after removing them from the visual field). For Piaget, this was the basis of thought because it demonstrates that infants can hold representations of objects in their minds.

Preoperational stage, 2–7 years

This stage is characterized by the development of conservation, where children can appreciate all the visual aspects of an object instead of just taking in one which can give incorrect responses in tests of conservation This is displayed with the pencils test—two identical pencils are placed so that they have their bases and tips aligned. One is then moved relative to the other so that one looks longer than the other (if one ignores the fact that the bases have moved relative to each other). Children who conserve will not infer that, when the pencils have moved, one must be longer than the other.

Concrete operational thought, 7–11 years

Children at this stage are capable of conservation but cannot undertake tasks involving abstract reasoning.

Formal operational thought, 11–15 years
At this stage the ability of abstract reasoning develops.

Language acquisition
The process of language acquisition is not well understood but the trend of thought (Chomsky, Pinker) has it that there is a preprogrammed way of understanding language (a 'deep grammar').

This inbuilt understanding of the workings of language allows rapid learning at a young age, no matter how that language is presented [i.e. learning and ease of use is the same for verbal and sign systems (deaf children learn sign language more quickly and use it in a far richer fashion than their hearing parents)].

Cognitive degeneration
The ageing brain
The gross changes in the brain include reductions in total volume, weight, and size of gyri, and an increase in ventricular size.

There are changes in the distribution of cell types. The number of cells in a given volume remains constant. There is, however, a steady decrease in the number of large neurons, accompanied by an increase in both small neurons and glial cells from the age of 20 years onwards.

There is a loss of intracortical myelin, which may be caused by loss of large pyramidal cells.

Neuronal death may be due to pre-programming, sensitivity to certain factors, or accumulated mutations.

Alterations in cellular structure include:
- Pyramidal cells in layer III of the frontal cortex anterior to the motor area develop swellings called meganeurites, possibly due to accumulation of cell debris.
- Pyramidal cells undergo atrophy of their dendritic arbor by losing dendritic spines, resulting in a loss of synaptic connections.

Successful ageing
The above structural changes need not cause loss of cognitive function if surviving neurons replace the lost synapses. Compensatory sprouting of dendrites by remaining neurons can maintain the total number of synaptic connections. This process is called reactive synaptogenesis.

Reactive synaptogenesis explains why there is an increase in the length of dendrites in hippocampal granule cells between middle and old age. The mean dendritic length begins to fall back after 80 years, suggesting that there is a limit to how long this process can continue protecting against the effects of cell loss.

Dementia
Dementia has emerged as a modern disease, owing to increases in life expectancy. Of individuals aged over 65 years, 5% are severely demented.

The most common form of dementia is the Alzheimer type, where there is a cognitive decline affecting all aspects of cognition and personality e.g. memory, attention, orientation, etc. The neuronal pathology is characteristic, including:
- Disturbances of the cytoskeleton, called neurofibrillary tangles, composed of paired helical filaments of a protein called τ (tau), which is an abnormally phosphorylated form of a microtubule-associated protein.
- Extracellular deposits of protein rich in β-amyloid and apolipoprotein E, called senile plaques. The precursor of β-amyloid is a cell membrane protein acting as a protease inhibitor. Mutations in the gene coding for the precursor protein may be responsible for some of the familial cases of Alzheimer's disease.

There is a characteristic decrease in brain weight and cortical atrophy. There is marked loss of neurons, usually most prominent in the hippocampus, parahippocampal gyrus, and the frontal, anterior temporal, and parietal cortices (mainly affecting glutamatergic pyramidal neurons). Cell loss also occurs in the nucleus basalis

Of the many causes of dementia, widespread cerebrovascular disease is one of the commonest. It is termed multi-infarct dementia, which progresses in a stepwise pattern as infarcts accumulate.

(diffuse acetylcholine projections throughout the forebrain) and there have been (largely unsuccessful) therapeutic strategies to increase acetylcholine release in the brain.

Psychological aspects of ageing

The normal changes in cognitive function begin at between 50 and 60 years of age and can be divided as follows:

- Reduction in the ability to perform problem-solving tasks, particularly if the problems are very novel or involve switching between different types of response.
- Slowing of responses in certain cognitive tests, due to reductions in decision speed rather than motor function.
- Memory function decreases, affecting visual information more than verbal information, and recall more than recognition.

Often there are changes in social functioning, so-called disengagement behaviour, where there is withdrawal from social contact. This may be caused by a lack of opportunity for social contact due to physical limitations on travel or financial limitations. As such, this may not represent a personality change.

Mood changes after the age of 60 typically include depression and anxiety as reactions against a perceived loss of a role in society, loss of social support, and bereavement.

- ○ **Give a rough outline of the cognitive ability of newborn babies and children, and of Piaget's theory of cognitive development.**
- ○ **Explain the macroscopic and microscopic structural changes in the ageing brain.**
- ○ **Explain why reactive synaptogenesis accounts for successful ageing.**
- ○ **Outline the psychological aspects of ageing.**

PHARMACOLOGY OF HIGHER CENTRAL NERVOUS SYSTEM FUNCTION

Anxiolytics and hypnotics

Anxiety is an exaggeration of a normal state with a cognitive component (unpleasant feelings of fear and restlessness) and a somatic component (tachycardia, gastrointestinal upset, sweating) due to autonomic activation. Anxiolytics reduce the symptoms of anxiety and hypnotics enable people to sleep, although this distinction is not clear-cut, particularly if anxiety is the main impediment to normal sleep.

Benzodiazepines

Benzodiazepines bind to γ-aminobutyric acid A (GABA$_A$) receptors (ligand-gated Cl$^-$ channels), increasing their affinity for GABA. This increases the inhibitory effect of GABA on the postsynaptic cell.

Benzodiazepines have four main actions:

- Anxiolysis (both the cognitive and somatic symptoms).
- Sedation and sleep.
- Anticonvulsant.
- Reduction in voluntary muscle tone.

Their clinical uses are in anxiety states, preoperative sedation, status epilepticus, acute alcohol withdrawal, and sedation during endoscopy and bronchoscopy.

Their main side effects are:

- Psychomotor impairment and drowsiness.
- Incoordination, weakness, diplopia.
- Amnesia.
- Aggression can be released from inhibition.
- Dependence.

Fig. 10.5 shows the mechanism and site of action of benzodiazepines.

Dependence is shown after 4–6 weeks and is both psychological and physical. The withdrawal syndrome (in 30% of patients) comprises rebound anxiety and insomnia, tremors, and twitching. Withdrawal is more severe after taking a short-acting benzodiazepine.

In overdose, benzodiazepines alone will produce a long sleep but, if alcohol is taken as well, the central nervous system depressant effects are potentiated and fatal respiratory depression can result. Treatment is with a benzodiazepine antagonist, flumazenil.

- Flumazenil antagonizes the effect of benzodiazepines (anxiolytic, anticonvulsant) and also antagonizes the effect of a class of drugs called β-carbolines (anxiogenic, proconvulsant). β-Carbolines therefore bind to the same receptor as benzodiazepines but they have opposing effects, possibly due to fluctuations in the conformational shape of the binding site and receptor function.
- As β-carbolines have the reverse effect of benzodiazepines and can have their effects blocked, they are called inverse agonists.

Fig. 10.6 outlines the differences between the benzodiazepines. Some have active metabolites with a half-life longer than that of the administered parent drug. This is important if the drug is taken for a long time, particularly in the elderly, as a prolonged sedated state could result.

5-Hydroxytryptamine modulators

- There is a 5-HT theory of anxiety that implicates altered functioning of the cortical innervation from the raphe nuclei. Essentially, high levels of 5-HT cause anxiety.
- The drive to develop drugs affecting the 5-HT systems is to find an anxiolytic drug that does not cause sedation and incoordination. Fig. 10.7 shows the mechanism of action of drugs acting at 5-HT synapses. The clinical efficacy of these drugs is still under review.

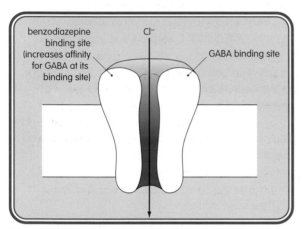

Fig. 10.5 Mechanism and site of action of benzodiazepines.

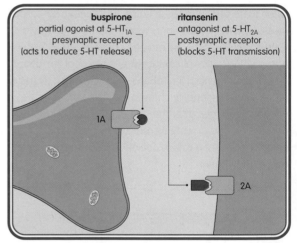

Fig. 10.7 Sites of action of anxiolytics modulating 5-HT transmission.

Fig. 10.6 Properties of benzodiazepines.

Properties of benzodiazepines			
Drug (half-life in brackets)	Metabolite (half-life in brackets)	Duration (h) of action	Clinical use
lorazepam (1–12 h)	none	12–18	anxiolysis, hypnosis
temazepam (8–12 h)	none	12–18	anxiolysis, hypnosis
diazepam (20–40 h)	nordiazepam (60 h)	24–28	anxiolysis, anticonvulsant
alprazolam (6–12 h)	hydroxylated metabolite (6 h)	24	anxiolysis

○ **What are the psychological and somatic symptoms of anxiety?**

○ **Relate the mode of action of the benzodiazepines to their clinical effectiveness.**

○ **What are the side effects of benzodiazepine use?**

○ **What is the rationale for using 5-HT-modulating drugs in anxiety?**

Antiepileptics

Epilepsy is a chronic disease with an unknown cause in 70% of cases, although known causes are tumours, head injury, alcoholism, and cerebrovascular accidents. It is characterized by seizures, where there is a rapid discharge of impulses in a localized collection of neurons, which can spread to other areas. The effect on the body depends on the location of the focus of abnormal signals.

- Involvement of the motor cortex will produce convulsions.
- Involvement of the brainstem can produce unconsciousness.

Seizures

Seizures are classified according to the focus and spread of the discharges.

- Focal seizures. A focus in the motor cortex can result in a jacksonian march, where repetitive jerky movements of muscles occur, spreading over the whole body. Typically, there is no loss of consciousness during the seizure.
- Secondary generalized seizures have a focus (often in the temporal lobe) and then spread to other areas.
- Generalized seizures do not have a recognizable focus and involve the whole brain, producing loss of consciousness presenting in two ways. It can occur as a tonic–clonic seizure (grand mal epilepsy), where an initial episode of extensor muscle rigidity is followed by violent jerky movements. Alternatively, it

can occur as absences (petit mal epilepsy), where patients suddenly stop what they are doing and are unaware of their environment for a few moments.

Phenytoin

Phenytoin reduces the spread of a seizure. Electroencephalogram recordings show that it does not stop the 'spiking' at a focus and so it does not prevent the onset of an epileptic discharge, but stops it from involving other areas.

It blocks voltage-gated Na^+ channels and has a higher affinity for channels in the inactivated state. This state is prolonged, preventing the channel from opening, which stops the neuron from firing rapidly. The block is use dependent as, at higher frequencies, more channels are cycling through the inactivated state. This allows selectivity of action, as the phenytoin block is more likely to occur in neurons in a seizure focus.

Oral absorption is variable and phenytoin is metabolized in the liver by an enzyme system that is saturated at therapeutic doses and, as such, shows dose-dependent kinetics. This means that, at certain doses, the serum concentration can rise rapidly to toxic levels as there is only a limited capacity to get rid of it. Because patients will vary in the doses that saturate their enzyme system, the therapeutic regime starts with low doses and then increases, with careful monitoring of serum phenytoin.

The side effects of phenytoin are:

- Vertigo and cerebellar signs—ataxia, dysarthria, nystagmus.
- At high doses, sedation and interference with cognitive functions.
- Collagen effects—Gum hypertrophy and coarsening of facial features.
- Allergic reactions—rash, hepatitis, lymphadenopathy.
- Haematological effects—megaloblastic anaemia.
- Endocrine effects—hirsutism.
- Teratogenesis—may cause congenital malformations (cleft palate).

Phenytoin has many drug interactions, mainly because it induces the hepatic P_{450} oxidase system, increasing the metabolism of oral contraceptives, anticoagulants, dexamethasone, and pethidine.

It is used for all types of epilepsy except absences.

Carbamazepine

The mechanism of action of carbamazepine is the same as for phenytoin.

It is well absorbed orally, with a long half-life (25–60 h) when first given.

Its side-effect profile is really limited to the nervous system, with ataxia, nystagmus, dysarthria, vertigo, and sedation. Like phenytoin, it is a strong enzyme inducer, causing similar interactions, and induces its own metabolism, which is why its half-life decreases if taken regularly.

It is used for all types of epilepsy except absences.

Valproate

Valproate has two mechanisms of action:
- As for phenytoin.
- It increases GABA content and GABA action, although this has no clear explanation.

It is well absorbed orally, has a half-life of 10–15 hours, and has much fewer side effects than other anticonvulsants, with the main problems being nausea, vomiting, and abdominal pain. Rarely, it can cause hepatitis and may be teratogenic. It interacts with other central nervous system depressants (e.g. alcohol), potentiating their effects.

It is used in all types of epilepsy, particularly absences.

Ethosuximide

The mechanism of action of ethosuximide is unknown. It is used only for absences, as it may make tonic–clonic attacks worse. Its side effects are nausea, loss of appetite, and mood swings.

Vigabatrin (γ-vinyl-GABA)

Vigabatrin is an irreversible inhibitor of GABA transaminase and so reduces the metabolism of GABA. This means that more GABA is available for release. It is used as an adjunct to other therapies that do not adequately control a patient's epilepsy.

Its side effects are drowsiness, dizziness, depression, and visual hallucinations, and it is contraindicated if patients have a history of psychiatric problems. Abrupt withdrawal leads to rebound seizures.

It is used in combination for all types of epilepsy except absences.

Phenobarbitone

Phenobarbitone is a barbiturate and has two anticonvulsant actions:
- It binds to the $GABA_A$ receptor, potentiating the effect of normal GABA release.
- It reduces glutamate-mediated excitation.

Its main side effect is sedation which, together with the fatal central nervous system depression it causes in overdose, limits its use clinically. It also causes cerebellar signs and is an enzyme inducer.

It is used for all types of epilepsy except absences.

Clonazepam

Clonazepam is a benzodiazepine and potentiates the normal effect of GABA binding.

Its side effects are sedation and a reduction in the anticonvulsant properties.

It is used intravenously in status epilepticus, where seizures occur constantly and can be fatal without intervention.

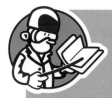

- Describe different types of epilepsy.
- Relate the action of phenytoin to its ability to stop seizure spread.
- State the actions and side effects of anticonvulsant drugs.

Drugs used in affective disorders

Affective disorders involve a disturbance of mood and can be thought of as pathological extremes along a normal continuum of mood change. They are classified according to which extremes they encompass and the type of symptoms that patients report.
- Unipolar affective disorders present either with mania (euphoria, increased motor activity, flight of ideas, and grandiose delusions) or depression (misery, malaise, and despair).
- Bipolar affective disorder involves swings between episodes of depression and mania.

Attempts have been made to classify types of depression, focusing on two clear groups of symptoms:

- 'Reactive' depression, where there is a clear psychological cause, involving less-severe symptoms and less likelihood of biological disturbance.
- 'Endogenous' depression, where there is no clear cause and more severe symptoms (e.g. suicidal thoughts) and greater likelihood of biological disturbance (e.g. sleep disturbance, anorexia, weight loss or gain). Depressions with some of these features tend to respond better to drug therapy.

Monoamine theory of depression

For many years it was thought that depression was due to reduced activity of monoamines (dopamine, noradrenaline). This theory explains why:

- Monoamine oxidase inhibitors can improve mood by reducing the metabolism of monoamines.
- Tricyclic antidepressants can improve mood by blocking the uptake of noradrenaline from the synaptic cleft.
- Reserpine produces depression by depleting monoaminergic nerve terminals.
- Methyldopa produces depression by inhibiting noradrenaline synthesis.

The theory cannot explain why:

- Amphetamine, cocaine, and L-dopa, which all affect monoamine systems, do not elevate the mood of depressed patients.
- Atypical antidepressants (e.g. iprindole) work without manipulating monoaminergic systems.
- There is a 'therapeutic' delay of 2 weeks between the full neurochemical effects of antidepressants and the start of their therapeutic effect.

It is unlikely that monoamine mechanisms alone are responsible for the symptoms of depression.

Tricyclic antidepressants (TCAs)

This class of drugs act by reducing the uptake of noradrenaline and 5-HT from the synaptic cleft. Examples are imipramine and amitriptyline and they have a similar efficacy.

The side-effect profile includes:

- Muscarinic blocking effects—dry mouth, blurred vision, constipation.

- α-Adrenergic blocking effects—postural hypotension.
- Noradrenaline uptake block in the heart, causing arrhythmia (greater with amitriptyline).
- Central effects—sedation (greater with amitriptyline), convulsions, mania.
- Weight gain.
- Interactions with alcohol and antihypertensive drugs.

In overdose, patients present with confusion, mania, and dysrhythmia.

The main use of TCAs is in depression with 'endogenous' features, and amitriptyline helps in disturbed sleep but is avoided if patients are apathetic. They also help in phobic disorders, obsessive–compulsive disorder and panic disorder.

Monoamine oxidase inhibitors (MAOIs)

MAO has two main forms, MAO_A and MAO_B, which differ in terms of substrate preference. Inhibition of the A form correlates best with antidepressant efficacy. These drugs reduce the activity of MAO, mainly affecting 5-HT and noradrenaline nerve terminals. Examples are phenelzine (irreversible inhibitor) and moclobemide (selective for MAO_A).

The side-effect profile includes:

- Interactions with indirectly acting amines, either tyramine in food (cheese, wine) or over-the-counter cold cures containing ephedrine or phenylephrine. Inhibition of MAO in the liver means that indirectly acting amines that would normally be metabolized can gain access to the systemic circulation. This causes noradrenaline release, resulting in large blood pressure increases and possibly death from a cerebrovascular accident.
- Central nervous system stimulation—excitement, tremor.
- Sympathetic blockade—hypotension.
- Muscarinic blockade—dry mouth, blurred vision, constipation.
- Phenelzine can be hepatotoxic.

In overdose, patients present with convulsions.

MAOIs are mainly used in severe depression, particularly moclobemide.

Selective serotonin reuptake inhibitors (SSRIs)

SSRIs are as effective as TCAs, suggesting that 5-HT mechanisms, rather than noradrenaline mechanisms, are partly responsible for depression. Examples are fluvoxamine and fluoxetine.

Their side-effect profile is much better than that of TCAs and MAOIs, as there are no amine interactions, anticholinergic actions, adrenergic blockade, or toxic effects in overdose; however, it includes:

- Nausea and headache.
- Insomnia.
- Rare serotonin syndrome of hyperthermia and cardiovascular collapse when used in conjunction with MAOIs.

SSRIs are now the most widely prescribed antidepressants.

Lithium

Given as lithium carbonate, it acts as a mood stabilizer with antimanic and antidepressant activity. It is restricted to treatment of bipolar disorder. Its mechanism of action is unclear but probably involves modulation of second-messenger pathways of cAMP and IP_3.

It has a very low therapeutic index and plasma lithium levels need to be monitored because of its severe side effects:

- Central nervous system—tremor, weakness, headache.
- Nausea and vomiting.
- Nephrogenic diabetes insipidus.
- Hypothyroidism.
- Oedema and weight gain.

In overdose, patients present with vomiting, diarrhoea, tremor, ataxia, and coma.

Atypical antidepressants

Examples are mianserin and iprindole. They have no common action and, for iprindole, no effect on amine mechanisms.

Overview

An overview of affective disorders is given in Fig. 10.8.

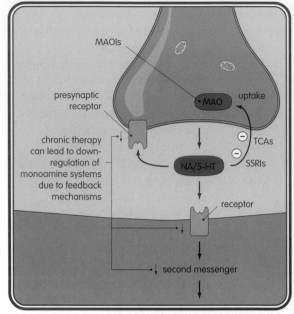

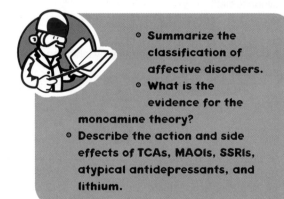

Fig. 10.8 Mechanism of action of antidepressants.

- Summarize the classification of affective disorders.
- What is the evidence for the monoamine theory?
- Describe the action and side effects of TCAs, MAOIs, SSRIs, atypical antidepressants, and lithium.

Antipsychotics (neuroleptics)

Antipsychotic drugs are used in the treatment of schizophrenia, which can be thought of as a collection of disordered thinking, perceiving, and behaving. Some symptoms tend to occur together, and different types of schizophrenia can be described according to this grouping:

- Positive symptoms (delusions, hallucinations, impaired reasoning).
- Negative symptoms (social withdrawal, lack of drive, behavioural disorders).

The presentation and pattern of illness is very variable. In general, the positive symptoms tend to occur acutely and then a chronic course develops, involving more of the negative symptoms.

Of the population, 1% have schizophrenia (a finding found across many cultures); in 75% of cases the onset is between 17 and 25 years and 64% of patients are men.

Theories of the cause of schizophrenia

A theory of the cause of schizophrenia must allow for genetic factors (monozygotic twins will both have schizophrenia in 50% of cases, dizygotic twins only in 17%) and environmental factors (stressful events often precede onset and influence the course of the illness).

The dopamine theory—increased dopamine transmission

- Evidence for—the clinical dose of an antipsychotic is proportional to its ability to block the D_2 receptor. PET ligand scans show that there are increased D_2 receptors in the nucleus accumbens. Psychiatric side effects are seen in drugs that increase dopaminergic transmission (L-dopa, amphetamine, bromocriptine).
- Evidence against—the level of dopamine metabolites in the cerebrospinal fluid of patients is normal or low. This suggests that dopamine is not the only factor causing symptoms.

The developmental theory—disordered development

- Evidence for—schizophrenic patients show reduced temporal lobe size compared with controls. Those born in winter months are more likely to develop schizophrenia, possibly because of viral infection of the mother before birth.
- Evidence against—not all studies agree on their findings and the theory does not explain the efficacy of neuroleptic drugs.

Neuroleptic side effects—dopamine pathways

There are three main dopamine pathways in the brain:

- Mesolimbic dopamine, running from the midbrain to the nucleus accumbens and amygdala, affecting thought and motivation.
- Nigrostriatal dopamine, running from the midbrain to the caudate nuclei, affecting motor control.
- Tubero-infundibular, running from the hypothalamus to the pituitary gland, regulating prolactin secretion.

The side-effect profile of neuroleptics is explained by:

- Disruption of the dopamine pathways.
- Blockade of muscarinic receptors.
- Blockade of α-receptors.

A summary of the profile is shown in Fig. 10.9.

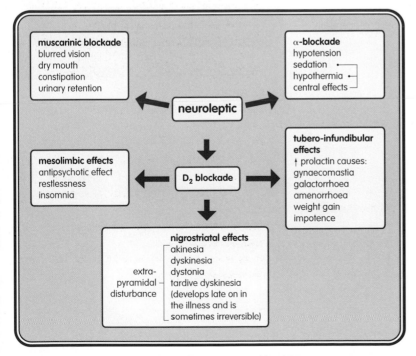

Fig. 10.9 Pharmacological effects of neuroleptic medication.

Phenothiazines

This class of compounds is split up into three groups by the side chain on the general formula producing different side-effect patterns:

- Aliphatic side chains (e.g. in chlorpromazine) produce strong sedation, a moderate muscarinic block, and moderate motor disturbance.
- Piperadine side chains (e.g. in thioridazine) produce moderate sedation, strong muscarinic block, and low motor disturbance.
- Piperazine side chains (e.g. in fluphenazine) produce low sedation, low muscarinic block, and strong motor disturbance.

Thioxanthines and butyrophenones

These two groups of compounds have the same profile of low sedation, low muscarinic blockade, and strong motor disturbance.

- Flupenthixol is a thioxanthine.
- Haloperidol is a butyrophenone.

Atypical neuroleptics

Drugs that have antipsychotic action but produce less intense motor side effects are termed 'atypical'.

Clozapine acts mainly on D_4 receptors and is often used in chronic cases that are resistant to other drugs. It has strong antimuscarinic activity, high prolactin-secreting ability, and is a sedative. The very minor effect on the motor system is because D_4 rather than D_2 receptors are preferentially blocked.

Overall neuroleptic side-effect profile

As well as the autonomic, endocrine, behavioural, and motor effects explained by clear disturbances of transmitter function, there are other effects:

- Toxic response. Agranulocytosis due to toxic bone marrow depression, particularly with clozapine. Cholestatic jaundice occurs in 2–4%. Skin rashes occur in 5% of patients.
- Ocular problems. Deposits in the cornea and lens occur with chlorpromazine and thioridazine.
- Malignant neuroleptic syndrome. An idiopathic response with fever, extrapyramidal motor disturbance, muscle rigidity, and coma.

- ○ Detail the different symptom patterns that schizophrenia can present. State the different theories of the cause of schizophrenia.
- ○ Relate the antipsychotic effect and side effects of neuroleptics to their dopaminergic, noradrenergic, and muscarinic blocking ability.
- ○ Name the classes and side effects of the neuroleptics.

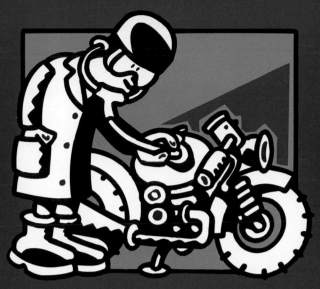

CLINICAL
ASSESSMENT

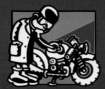

11. Taking a History

THINGS TO REMEMBER WHEN TAKING A HISTORY

Taking a history is probably the most important part of assessment of the patient with neurological symptoms.

Observation of the patients as they walk into the examination room or as you approach the bed is all-important.

- Do they appear unwell?
- Do they use walking aids (sticks, crutches, frame, wheelchair, callipers)?
- Do they appear to be independent, or clearly need help from others?
- Are there any obvious morphological abnormalities (e.g. weakness on one side, drooping of the face, wasting of the muscles)?

- Introduce yourself.
- Explain who you are.
- Ask if you may talk to and examine them.
- Ask their age and occupation.
- Ask whether they are right- or left-handed—if you don't ask this at the beginning, you will forget about it until your consultant asks you!

In hospital, general observation of the patient's environment is always important.

- Notice the sputum pot and diabetic urine-tests.
- Cards and flowers from friends and relatives may indicate a supportive home network.

Immediately, you will observe important points regarding their neurological status.

- Do they respond appropriately (indicating probable preservation of important higher mental functioning)?
- Do they appear to be depressed (which may be part of their neurological condition or may indicate a reaction to it)?
- Do they appear to be elated (again, a feature of some neurological illnesses such as multiple sclerosis)?
- Is their speech normal?
- You may notice additional features such as tremor, agitation, twitches, and abnormal movements.

Do not worry about what may be causing these at this stage, as things will become much clearer as you progress through a systematic history-taking process.

Neurological symptoms
Remember these by working from the 'head down':
- Headache
- Memory problems
- Speech difficulty
- Dizzy turns
- Swallowing
- Weakness
- Numbness
- Bladder or bowel disturbance
- Walking difficulty

THE STRUCTURE OF THE HISTORY

The complaint

From the patient's point of view. Ask:

- 'What is the main problem?'
- 'What was it that caused you to go to your doctor/come to the hospital?'

When presenting the history to others, use the patient's language (e.g. 'This woman complains of seeing double' rather than 'This woman has horizontal diplopia').

The history of the presenting complaint (HPC):

- When was it first noted by the patient?
- Has it worsened, improved, or stayed the same since?
- What is its nature (e.g. headache may be sharp, dull, an ache, a throb, etc.)?
- Is there anything that makes it better (e.g. medicines, sleep, exercise) or worse (e.g. time of day, posture, exercise)?

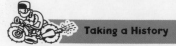

- Have any other symptoms developed since this first complaint was noticed (e.g. main complaint may be weakness of the hand, but a numb patch may have developed more recently)?
- Have any tests already been performed, and if so where and by whom?
- Has the patient ever had other neurological symptoms in the past (these may be related, e.g. an episode of transient visual loss 5 years previously in a young woman now complaining of difficulty in walking)?
- It is often worth running through a checklist of neurological symptoms (hints and tips).

Review of systems (ROS)

- Gastrointestinal: appetite, weight loss/gain, swallowing, bowel function (change ?).
- Cardiovascular: chest pain, breathlessness, claudication.
- Respiratory: cough, breathlessness.
- Genitourinary: bladder function, impotence, sexual function.
- Musculoskeletal: joint pain, stiffness.

Past medical history (PMH)

- Any serious illnesses in the past or intercurrently (e.g. diabetes, hypertension, tumour)?

Drug history (DH)

- Is the patient taking any medicines now, or have any been taken for some time in the past?
- Are there any known drug allergies?

Family history (FH)

- Are there any 'family illnesses'? Are parents, siblings, and children alive and well, and if not, what did they die from and at what age? *Draw* a family tree (Fig. 11.1).

Social history

- Home circumstances: own home, stairs, social-service help.
- Smoking (ever).
- Alcohol (ever heavy consumption).
- Diet (vegetarian or vegan).
- Heterosexual or homosexual.

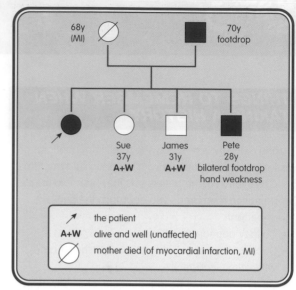

Fig. 11.1 The Lane family: autosomal dominant hereditary sensory motor neuropathy.

Summary

When presenting the history, run through the categories described above, always starting with the same pattern (e.g. 'Miss Randolph is a 40-year-old right-handed administrator who complains of numbness in the feet').

Describe the history of the HPC, PMH, and ROS. You do not have to mention specifically all negative points, but it is worth pointing out those that are important (e.g. 'She has no history of diabetes').

Say whether the patient is taking any medication.

Describe the family history, if relevant; if not, explain that 'there is no relevant family history'.

Describe important social points (e.g. 'she drinks only moderate alcohol and has never smoked').

You will then move on to your examination findings.

When presenting the history, always start with the same sequence:
- **Name**
- **Age**
- **Handedness**
- **Occupation**
- **Complaint** (in the patient's words)

COMMON PRESENTING COMPLAINTS

In this section, differential diagnoses are given for the following common conditions or complaints: headache, central nervous system infection, dementia, numbness and tingling, dizziness, gait disturbances, weakness, coma, sudden onset of hemiparesis, and seizures.

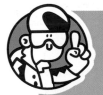

The most common causes of each complaint are indicated by asterisks.

You should consider these first.

Headache
Differential diagnosis (Fig. 11.2)

- Migraine*
- Tension/stress headache*
- Chronic daily headache*
- Cluster headache
- Hypertension
- Increased intracranial pressure (ICP) (space-occupying lesion, SOL; cerebral vein thrombosis).
- Infection (meningitis, abscess, postherpetic neuralgia)
- Trauma (head injury, subdural haematoma).
- Vascular (intracerebral haemorrhage, subarachnoid haemorrhage)
- Drug/toxin-related (vasodilators, caffeine withdrawal, carbon monoxide exposure)

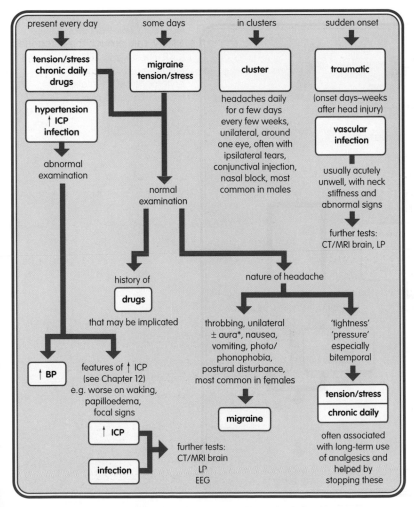

Fig. 11.2 Headache algorithm. *Migrainous auras are transient focal cerebral or brainstem symptoms that accompany the headache (e.g. visual—especially scintillating scotomata; flickering lights in homonomous field). (EEG, electroencephalogram; ICP, intracranial pressure; LP, lumbar puncture.)

Central nervous system infections
Differential diagnosis (Fig. 11.3)

This is not strictly a 'presenting complaint' but is an important cause of a group of presenting features, as shown in Fig. 11.3.

The list of organisms that may cause CNS infection is huge. The following are important.

Meningitis

- Viral* [coxsackievirus, echovirus, Epstein–Barr virus, herpes simplex virus, paramyxovirus (mumps), human immunodeficiency virus]
- Bacterial* ['the big 3': **NHS**; **N**eisseria meningitidis (meningococcus), **H**aemophilus influenzae, **S**treptococcus pneumoniae (pneumococcus); Staphylococcus aureus, Escherichia coli, Listeria monocytogenes]
- Fungal (Cryptococcus, Histoplasma, Aspergillus)

Encephalitis

- Viral [herpes simplex virus* primarily, causes of meningitis, varicella-zoster virus (chickenpox), cytomegalovirus, measles virus, influenza virus]
- Postviral [measles—subacute sclerosing panencephalomyelitis (SSPE)]

Other

- Cerebral abscess (Streptococcus pneumoniae, Staphylococcus aureus, Streptococcus milleri, Cryptococcus, Toxoplasma, Cysticercosis, Hydatid, Entamoeba)
- Subdural empyema/abscess (Streptococcus pneumoniae, S. milleri, Staphylococcus aureus).
- Transverse myelitis (Mycoplasma pneumoniae, tuberculosis, Borrelia, coxsackievirus, echovirus, herpes simplex virus, varicella-zoster virus, human immunodeficiency virus)

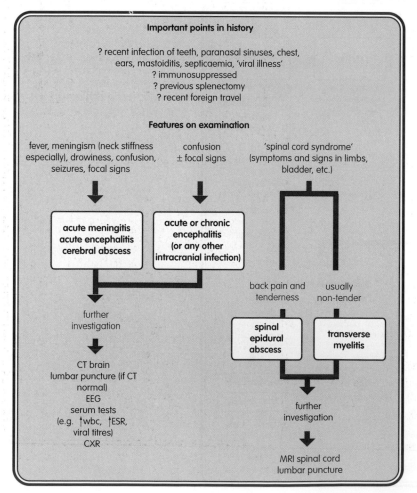

Fig. 11.3 Central nervous system infection algorithm. (CXR, chest X-ray; EEG, electroencephalogram; ESR, erythrocyte sedimentation rate; wbc, white blood cells.)

- Spinal epidural abscess *(Staphylococcus aureus, Streptococcus pyogenes, Pseudomonas).*

Common opportunistic infections
- Fungal: *Cryptococcus*
- Protozoan: *Toxoplasma*
- Viral: cytomegalovirus, varicella-zoster virus (especially shingles)
- Other: PML (progressive multifocal leucoencephalopathy, associated with JC virus)

Dementia
Differential diagnosis (Fig. 11.4)
Again, not in itself a 'presenting complaint' of the patient but an important clinical presentation with many underlying causes.

The surgical sieve, as outlined below, will enable you to remember all the causes of this, but it is more sensible to relate them in approximate order of likelihood (i.e. think of the asterisked causes first).

Congenital
- Huntington's disease
- Presenile dementia
- Adrenoleucodystrophy
- Canavan's disease
- Metachromatic leucodystrophy
- GM1 gangliosidosis

Acquired
- Degenerative: Alzheimer's disease*, Pick's disease, Parkinson's disease, Lewy body disease
- Inflammatory: multiple sclerosis
- Vascular: multi-infarct dementia*
- Infective: human immunodeficiency virus, syphilis, Creutzfeldt–Jakob disease, postencephalitis/postmeningitis, progressive multifocal leucoencephalopathy, Whipple's disease
- Endocrine: hypo*/hyperthyroidism
- Metabolic: B_{12} deficiency*, see congenital causes, organ failure, anoxia
- Iatrogenic: drug-induced*; sedatives
- Idiopathic: normal pressure hydrocephalus (NPH)
- Neoplastic: intracranial tumour (benign/malignant, primary/secondary), paraneoplastic
- Psychological: depression*
- Traumatic: head injury, subdural haematoma
- Toxic: chronic alcoholism

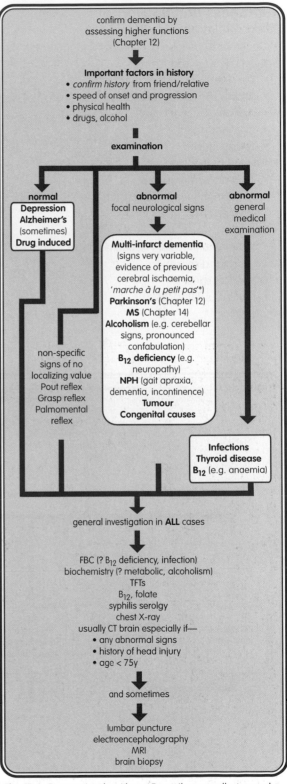

Fig. 11.4 Dementia algorithm. *Describes small-stepped gait typical of (but not specific to) multi-infarct disease. (TFTs, thyroid function tests.)

Numbness and tingling
Differential diagnosis (Fig. 11.5)
- Generalized peripheral neuropathy (Chapter 15). The most common causes are:
  - Diabetes*: by far the commonest
  - Vitamin B_{12} and B_1 deficiency
  - Alcohol
  - Carcinomatous
  - Drug-induced
- Isolated mononeuropathy:
  - Trauma/compression
  - Multiple mononeuropathy (Chapter 15, Hints and Tips, p. 213)
- Vascular:
  - Ischaemia (transient ischaemic attack, peripheral vascular disease)
- Other CNS causes:
  - Multiple sclerosis (MS)
- Idiopathic*

Dizziness
A very common complaint in neurological practice. Patients may use the term dizziness to describe a wide variety of sensations, including vertigo (a subjective sensation of movement, usually spinning), syncope (faintness and light-headedness caused by decrease in cerebral blood flow), fitting, confusion, nausea, headache, numbness, or tiredness. Be aware of this and check what the patient is describing.

Most commonly, dizziness describes episodes of either vertigo or syncope. A 'funny turn' in neurological practice is usually either one of these or is epileptic in nature.

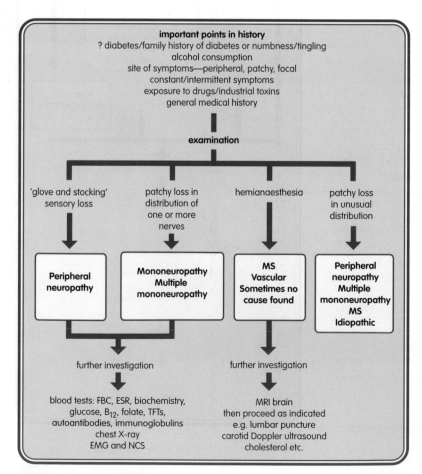

Fig. 11.5 Numbness and tingling algorithm.
(EMG, electromyogram; ESR, erythrocyte sedimentation rate; FBC, full blood count; NCS, nerve conduction studies; TFTs, thyroid function tests.)

Differential diagnosis (Fig. 11.6)
Vertigo
- Peripheral (inner ear)
  - Benign paroxysmal positional vertigo*
  - Benign recurrent vertigo
  - Vestibular neuronitis (also described as peripheral vestibulopathy, or viral labyrinthitis)*
  - Ménière's syndrome*
  - Infection
  - Head injury
  - Drugs (e.g. aminoglycosides)
- Central (in the brainstem or cranial nerve VIII)
  - Multiple sclerosis*
  - Brainstem ischaemia
- Basilar migraine
- Cerebellopontine angle (CPA) tumours

Syncope
- Simple faint (vasovagal attack)*
- Hypotension, especially postural* (drugs, dehydration, pregnancy, cardiac)
- Transient ischaemic attack* (carotid disease, cardioembolism)*
- Cardiac arrhythmia*
- Syncope induced by micturition, cough, straining, cold foods (ice-cream syncope)

Epilepsy (see Seizures, p. 135; see also Chapter 14, p. 204)

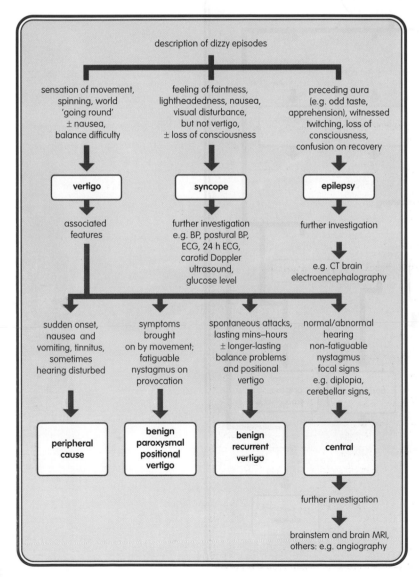

Fig. 11.6 Dizziness algorithm.

Gait disturbances
Differential diagnosis (Fig. 11.7)
Weakness

- Upper motor neuron
  - Hemiparesis (stroke*, cerebral tumour, multiple sclerosis), paraparesis (multiple sclerosis*, spinal cord infarction, tumour, cord compression, midline meningioma)
- Lower motor neuron (footdrop*, spinal claudication, root disease)

Ataxia

- Cerebellar disease
- Proprioceptive loss (peripheral neuropathy)

Extrapyramidal disease

- Parkinson's disease*
- Other extrapyramidal disorders

Apraxia

- Normal pressure hydrocephalus
- *Marche à la petit pas* of multi-infarct disease

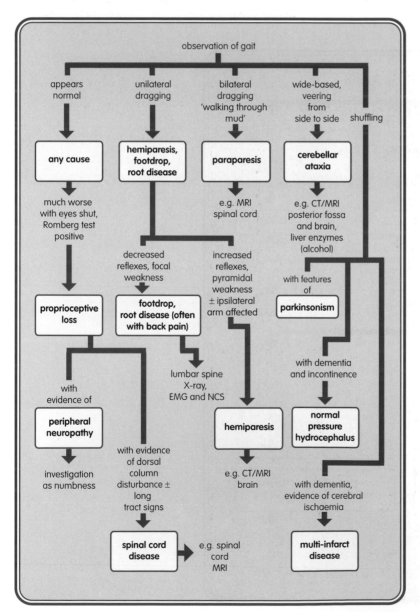

Fig. 11.7 Gait disturbance algorithm. (EMG, electromyogram; NCS, nerve conduction studies.)

Weakness
Differential diagnosis (Fig. 11.8)

This is best considered from an anatomical point of view, starting at the 'top' of the motor tracts and working down. Simple causes are given for each, but you should be able to add to these without difficulty.

- Upper motor neuron
  - Cortex/cerebral hemispheres (cerebrovascular accident, tumour)
  - Brainstem/cerebellar connections (multiple sclerosis, tumour)
- Spinal cord
  - Compression, ischaemia, tumour, multiple sclerosis
- Lower motor neuron
  - Anterior horn cell (motor neuron disease)
  - Nerve root (disc protrusion)
  - Peripheral nerve (diabetic neuropathy)
- Muscle
  - Neuromuscular junction (myasthenia gravis)
  - Muscle (muscular dystrophy, polymyositis)
- 'Non-neurological'
  - Thyroid disorders (hypothyroidism/hyperthyroidism)
  - Malnutrition/dehydration
  - Cachexia (underlying carcinoma)
  - Electrolyte disturbances (hyponatraemia, hypernatraemia, hypokalaemia, hyperkalaemia)
  - Pain/stiffness caused by joint disease (arthritis)

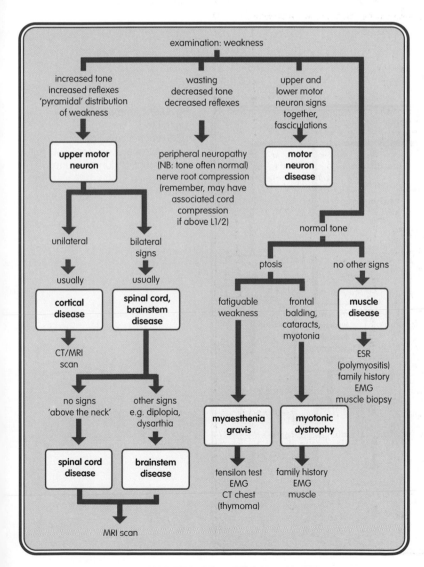

Fig. 11.8 Weakness algorithm. (EMG, electromyogram; ESR, erythrocyte sedimentation rate.)

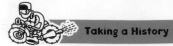

Coma
Differential diagnosis (Fig. 11.9)

- Intracranial
  - Infection* (meningitis, encephalitis, abscess, malaria, see Chapter 12)
  - Tumour
  - Cerebrovascular accident* (haemorrhage more commonly than infarction, subarachnoid haemorrhage)
  - Anoxic brain injury (following cardiac arrest, head injury, anaesthetic accident, respiratory failure)
  - Head injury*
- Metabolic
  - Hypoglycaemia*
  - Diabetic coma* (ketoacidosis, non-ketotic hyperglycaemia)
  - Liver failure
  - Renal failure
- Addison's disease, Cushing's disease
- Hypopituitarism
- Hyperammonaemia (liver failure, amino acid disorders, sodium valproate)
- Toxic
  - Drug-induced* (including drugs of abuse; heroin, Ecstasy, benzodiazepines, and overdose* of most medications)
  - Alcohol (excess, Wernicke's encephalopathy)
  - Carbon monoxide
- Hypothermia

Conditions that may mimic coma

- Akinetic mutism (persistent vegetative state)
- Locked-in syndrome
- Non-convulsive status epilepticus
- Catatonia

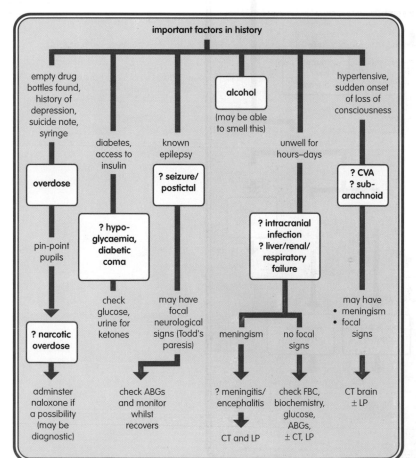

Fig. 11.9 Coma diagnostic algorithm.
(ABG, arterial blood gases; CVA, cerebrovascular accident; FBC, full blood count; LP, lumbar puncture.)

Sudden onset of hemiparesis
Differential diagnosis
Stroke is most likely and may be caused by any of the following:

- Atherothrombotic carotid disease* (predisposing factors—family history, smoking, hypertension, diabetes)
- Cardioembolic disease* (atrial fibrillation, AF; cardiac valve disease)
- Cardiac arrhythmia*
- Hyperviscosity syndrome (multiple myeloma, Waldenström's macroglobulinaemia, leukaemia)
- Hypotensive episode (watershed infarcts)

However, the differential diagnosis of a patient presenting with sudden collapse with or without focal neurological signs also includes:

- Epilepsy (see below; see also Chapter 14)

- Syncope (see above)
- Most of the causes of coma, especially:
  - Hypoglycaemia
  - Cerebral tumour
  - Subarachnoid haemorrhage

Seizures (see Chapter 14)
Differential diagnosis (Fig. 11.10)

- Primary generalized epilepsy*
- Secondary generalized epilepsy
- Partial (focal) seizures*
  - Simple (no impairment of consciousness)
  - Complex (with impairment of consciousness)
- Seizures due to focal structural (tumour, stroke*, infection, trauma) or metabolic (hypoglycaemia*; liver failure; drugs*, including overdose; toxins, especially alcohol and alcohol withdrawal*)

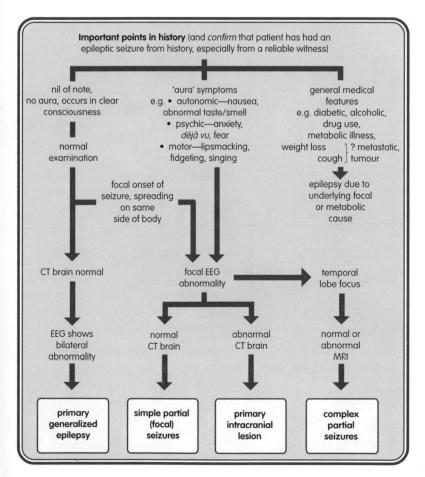

Fig. 11.10 Seizures diagnostic algorithm.
(EEG, electroencephalogram.)

- Outline the important features of the history of a 65-year-old man presenting with confusion.
- How would you approach the management of a 30-year-old woman who complains of a 1-year history of frontal headache?
- A 50-year-old man has been having dizzy spells for a month. What would you do?
- Outline your management of a 20-year-old man who presents to an Accident and Emergency Department unconscious.

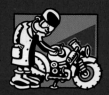
SPEECH

Speech production is organized at three levels: phonation, articulation, and language production.

Phonation

Phonation is the production of sounds as the air passes through the vocal cords. A disorder of this process is called dysphonia.

Assessment

Speech will have already been heard during the history taking, but if not, get the patient to talk by asking him or her any question. In dysphonia the speech volume is reduced and the voice sounds rather husky. Dysphonia is usually due to lesions of the recurrent laryngeal nerves, or to respiratory muscle weakness (e.g. Guillain–Barré syndrome)

Articulation

Articulation is the manipulation of sound as it passes through the upper airways by the palate, the tongue, and the lips to produce phonemes. A disorder of this process is called dysarthria.

Assessment

To assess articulation, ask the patient to repeat 'British Constitution', 'baby hippopotamus', and 'West Register street'. If the speech articulation is abnormal, this could be caused by:

- Cerebellar dysarthria: speech is slurred (sounds like a drunk), with 'staccato' or scanning quality.
- Extrapyramidal dysarthria: speech is soft and monotonous.
- Pseudobulbar dysarthria (see Fig. 12.28): speech is high pitched with a 'strangulated' quality and sounds like 'Donald Duck' speech.
- Bulbar dysarthria (see Fig. 12.28): speech has a nasal quality that may worsen as the patient continues to speak (suggesting myasthenia gravis).

Language production

Language production is the organization of phonemes into words and sentences, and is controlled by the speech centres in the dominant hemisphere. A disorder of this process is called dysphasia.

Assessment

To assess language production:

- Establish the patient's handedness. Dysphasia is a feature of dominant hemisphere dysfunction.
- Listen to the patient's spontaneous speech, assessing its fluency and contents.
- Assess the patient's comprehension by observing his or her response to simple commands: 'Open your mouth, look up to the ceiling'.
- Assess the patient's ability to name objects. Use your wrist-watch (face, hands, strap, buckle).
- Assess the patient's ability to repeat sentences: 'No ifs, ands, or buts'.
- If any of these features is abnormal, the patient is dysphasic.

Cerebrovascular disease and brain tumours are the commonest causes of dysphasia. Dysphasia is classified according to speech fluency and content, comprehension, and anatomical location of the lesions (Figs 12.1 and 12.2).

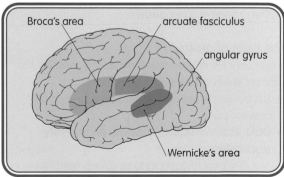

Fig. 12.1 Broca's and Wernicke's areas and their connecting arcuate fasciculus.

Classification of dysphasia					
Type	Lesion	Speech fluency	Speech content	Comprehension	Repetition
expressive	Broca's area	non-fluent	normal	normal	variable
anomic	angular gyrus	fluent	normal	normal	normal
receptive	Wernicke's area	fluent	impaired	impaired	variable
conductive	arcuate fasciculus	fluent	normal	normal	impaired
global	parietal lobe	non-fluent	impaired	impaired	impaired

Fig. 12.2 Classification of dysphasia.

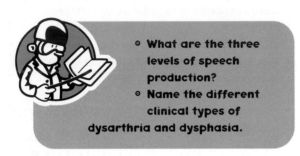

- **What are the three levels of speech production?**
- **Name the different clinical types of dysarthria and dysphasia.**

MENTAL STATE AND HIGHER FUNCTIONS

Consciousness

Consciousness is the state of being aware of self and the environment. It has two components:
- The level of arousal.
- The content of consciousness.

The level of arousal

A number of ill-defined terms are used to describe the different levels of arousal:
- Full awakefulness and responsiveness—normal arousal status.
- Obtundation—patient is drowsy and not fully responsive.
- Stupor—patient appears to be asleep, with little or no spontaneous activity; however, he or she is rousable when stimulated.
- Coma—patient is unresponsive and unrousable.

This aspect of consciousness is conventionally assessed using the Glasgow coma scale (see Fig. 12.39).

The content of consciousness

The content of consciousness is dependent on the patient's level of cognitive functioning. The content of consciousness can be assessed only when a reasonable degree of arousal is present. This aspect of consciousness is conventionally assessed using the mini-mental state examination (see later).

Appearance and behaviour

Assessment of the patient's mental state begins as soon as you meet him or her. The physical appearance can be helpful. Demented patients may look bewildered but unconcerned, or apathetic and withdrawn. Look for evidence of self-neglect, which is often concealed by relatives. Observe the patient's response to your questions during the history-taking, assessing his or her comprehension and whether he or she retains insight into his or her problem.

Affect

Ask the patient if he or she has been feeling anxious, depressed, or irritable, and decide if his or her mood is appropriate. Euphoric and manic patients look inappropriately cheerful and energetic, and tend to ignore or play down their problems and disabilities. Patients with emotional lability have sudden unprovoked outbursts of laughing or crying, which can be very distressing to them.

In cognitive impairment, patients' emotional reactions vary according to the severity of their illness:
- At the early stages, anxiety and depression might result from preserved insight into the increasing intellectual difficulties.
- In advanced stages, a flattening of the affect becomes apparent.

Attention and orientation

Attention

Ensure that the patient's comprehension is normal. Formal assessment of attention is done using serial reversals:

- 'Can you spell 'world' backwards for me, please'.
- 'Can you name the months of the year backwards, starting with December'.
- 'Can you count backwards from 20'.

Orientation

Assess the patient's orientation in time, place, and person. To test the patient's orientation in time, ask:

- 'What day of the week is it today?'
- 'How long have you been in hospital?'

To test the patient's orientation in place, ask:

- 'Can you tell me where are you now?'
- 'What city are we in?'

To test the patient's orientation in person, ask:

- 'Who is this person?' (point to a family member, a nurse, or a doctor).

Memory

Immediate memory (recall)

Establish that the patient's comprehension and attention are normal. Immediate recall is tested with digit span: 'Can you repeat these numbers after me, please'. Start with two or three figures, avoiding recognizable sequences. A normal individual can repeat a five- to seven-digit sequence.

Recent memory

Ask the patient about recent political, social, or sporting events, taking into account his or her premorbid intelligence and socio-economic status.

Ask the patient to memorize a short address (four or five words). Ask him or her to repeat the address after you to ensure that it has been registered. Distract the patient for the next 10 minutes (by continuing your assessment of his or her mental status), then ask him or her to repeat the address. Most normal individuals will be able to recall all the data in 10 minutes.

Visual memory can be tested by displaying a drawing for 5 seconds and asking the patient to redraw the design 10 seconds later (Fig. 12.3). Patients with visuospatial disorders will have difficulty with the task, even if their visual memory is intact.

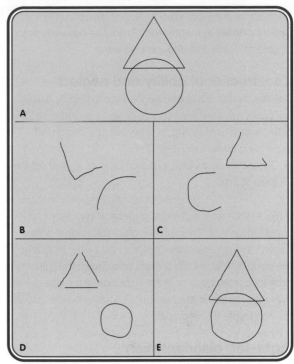

Fig. 12.3 Visual memory test showing (A) the standard design and (B–E) reproductions scored from 0–3.

Remote memory

Ask the patient about childhood, schooling, work history, or marriage. The accuracy of his or her answers should be verified by a relative.

Immediate and recent memory is usually affected early in dementia. However, remote memory is relatively spared in patients with minor degrees of brain damage, but is always affected in those with advanced dementia.

Calculation

This should be tested in the light of the patient's education. Give the patient simple addition or subtraction sums. Serial sevens or threes (subtracting sevens or threes serially from 100) is a useful test.

Dyscalculia is a prominent feature of Gerstmann's syndrome (dyscalculia, right–left disorientation, and finger agnosia), caused by dominant parietal lobe lesions.

Abstract thinking

This is tested by asking the patient to interpret common proverbs:

- 'A bird in the hand is worth two in the bush'.
- 'People in glass houses should not throw stones'.

Abstract thinking can also be tested by assessing the patient's ability to identify the similarities between pairs of objects: 'cow and dog, air and water'.

Constructional ability and neglect

Constructional ability and neglect are tested by asking the patient to construct simple designs (triangle, square) using match-sticks, and to draw or copy designs of increasing complexity (Fig. 12.4):

- 'Please draw a clock, put the hours on it, and set the time at 3:00'.

Patients with non-dominant parietal lesions have poor constructional ability (which is often associated with neglect to the contralateral side of the body, including the visual fields), which is often reflected in the patients' drawings (they copy only the right side of the design, or they draw and put the numbers on the one side, usually the right side, of the clock).

Right–left disorientation

Establish that the patient's comprehension is normal. Right–left disorientation is assessed by giving the patient simple commands of increasing complexity:

- 'Show me your right hand'.
- 'Put your left hand on your right ear'.

Right–left disorientation is seen in patients with dominant parietal lobe lesions.

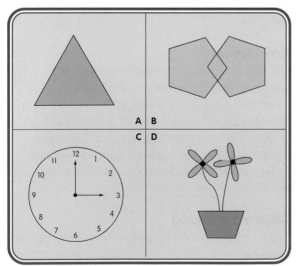

Fig. 12.4 Constructional tests drawings of increasing complexity to be reproduced by the patient.

Dyspraxia

Dyspraxia is the inability to perform a skilled movement in the absence of weakness, incoordination, sensory loss, or abnormal comprehension. Dyspraxia can be confined to the limbs, the trunk, or the buccofacial musculature.

Dyspraxia is tested by asking the patient to carry out particular tasks of increasing complexity:

- 'Stick out your tongue'.
- 'Pretend to whistle'.
- 'Show me how to use a toothbrush'.
- 'Show me how to take the cap off a toothpaste tube and squeeze the toothpaste onto a brush'.

There are some special forms of dyspraxia:

- Dressing dyspraxia.
- Constructional dyspraxia.
- Gait dyspraxia.

Agnosia

Agnosia is the inability to recognize a sensory input in the absence of primary sensory pathway dysfunction. It can affect a certain sensory modality in a global fashion (visual agnosia, auditory agnosia), or can affect a specific class of stimuli (colour agnosia).

Agnosia is tested by showing the patient a few objects and asking him or her to name each one. Allow the patient to manipulate the objects, which might improve recognition (by allowing him or her to use a different sensory input). Assess other sensory modalities:

- Auditory agnosia (inability to recognize sounds).
- Tactile agnosia (inability to recognize objects placed in the hand: astereognosis).
- Finger agnosia (inability to name fingers).
- Topographic agnosia (inability to comprehend three-dimensional sense).

Mini-mental state examination

It is often difficult to perform an extensive testing of higher cortical functions in every patient. Screening tests have been devised to allow rapid assessment. The mini-mental state examination (Fig 12.5) is one of many such tests. This is a helpful screening test, but has its limitations.

- The maximum score is 30.
- Scores 28–30 do not support the diagnosis of dementia.
- Scores 25–27 are borderline.
- Scores <25 are suggestive of dementia (if acute confusional state and depression are unlikely).

Cortical and subcortical dementia

Learn to differentiate between the features of cortical and subcortical dementia (Fig. 12.6). Patients with cortical dementia retain the ability to answer questions at a relatively normal speed. However, their answers are irrelevant and 'hopeless'.

- Q. How many arms do you have?
- A. Oh, not many!

Patients with subcortical dementia have difficulty in retrieving memories and their response time is therefore long. They are not totally 'hopeless' and often find the right answer with some help.

- Q. Who is the Prime Minister?
- A. Erm . . . I don't know.
- Q. Is it Bill Clinton, John Major, or Tony Blair?
- A: Tony Blair.

Clinical syndromes associated with specific focal hemispheric dysfunction
Frontal lobe

Conditions associated with frontal lobe dysfunction are:

- Altered personality, altered mood, loss of interest, loss of initiative.
- Expressive dysphasia (dominant hemisphere), and dyspraxia.

Fig. 12.5 The mini-mental state test.

Mini-mental state examination

Orientation
1. What is the year, season, date, month, day? (one point for each correct answer)
2. Where are we? Country, county, town, hospital, floor? (one point for each answer)

Registration
3. Name three objects, taking 1 second to say each. Then ask the patient all three once you have said them. One point for each correct answer. Repeat the questions until the patient learns all three

Attention and calculation
4. Serial sevens. One point for each correct answer. Stop after five answers.
   Alternative: spell 'words' backwards

Recall
5. Ask for names of three objects asked in question 3. One point for each correct answer

Language
6. Point to a pencil and a watch. Ask the patient to name them for you. One point for each correct answer
7. Ask the patient to repeat 'No ifs, ands, or buts'. One point
8. Ask the patient to follow a three-stage command: 'Take the paper in your right hand; fold the paper in half; put the paper on the floor.' Three points
9. Ask the patient to read and obey the following: CLOSE YOUR EYES. (Write this in large letters). One point
10. Ask the patient to write a sentence of his or her own choice. (The sentence must contain a subject and an object and make some sense.) Ignore spelling errors when scoring. One point
11. Ask the patient to copy two intersecting pentagons with equal sides (Fig 12.4B). Give one point if all the sides and angles are preserved, and if the intersecting sides from a quadrangle

Maximum score = 30 points

Features of cortical and subcortical dementia

	Example	Cognition	Insight	Memory	Response time	Personality	Mood
cortical dementia	Alzheimer's disease, Pick's disease	severely disturbed	absent	difficulty learning new information	normal	unconcerned	may be depressed
subcortical dementia	Parkinson's disease, Huntington's chorea	impaired problem solving	partially retained	difficulty retrieving learned information	slow	apathetic	often depressed

Fig. 12.6 Features of cortical and subcortical dementia.

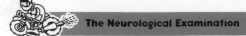

- Hemiparesis and primitive reflexes.
- Sphincter incontinence (bifrontal lesions).

Parietal lobe

Conditions associated with parietal lobe dysfunction on the dominant side are:

- Dysphasia, dyslexia, dysgraphia.
- Dyscalculia.
- Right–left disorientation.
- Finger agnosia.

Conditions associated with dysfunction of the non-dominant side are:

- Neglect to the contralateral side of the body.
- Constructional and dressing dyspraxia.
- Topographic agnosia.

Conditions associated with dysfunction of the non-dominant or dominant side are:

- Hemisensory disturbance or inattention.
- Lower quadrant homonymous field defect.

Temporal lobe

Conditions associated with temporal lobe dysfunction are:

- Amnesic syndromes.
- Dysphasia (dominant lobe).
- Upper quadrant homonymous field defect.

- **Describe the two components of consciousness.**
- **How would you assess a patient's attention, orientation, memory, calculation, and abstraction abilities? How would you test for agnosia and dyspraxia?**
- **Summarize the mini-mental state examination.**
- **List the differences between cortical and subcortical dementia.**

Occipital lobe

Conditions associated with occipital lobe dysfunction are:

- Visual field defects.
- Distortion of vision.
- Impaired visual recognition (visual agnosia).

GAIT

In normal gait, the erect moving body is supported by one leg at a time while the other swings forward in preparation for the next support move. Only one foot will be on the floor at any time, although both the heel of the anterior foot and the toes of the posterior foot will be on the ground momentarily when the body weight is transferred from one leg to the other. Normal gait requires input from the motor, sensory, cerebellar, and vestibular systems.

Assessment

The gait of a patient is assessed as follows:

- Ask the patient to walk up and down the examination room in his or her usual fashion, with his or her arms loose by his or her side.
- Observe the patient's posture, the pattern of his or her arm and leg movements, and the control of his or her trunk.
- If gait appears normal, ask the patient to heel–toe walk ('I would like you to walk heel to toe as if you are walking on a tightrope'). Walk alongside the patient to support him or her if he or she appears unsteady.
- If gait appears abnormal, classify it into one of the following patterns:

Hemiplegic gait

Hemiplegic gait (Fig. 12.7A) is caused by unilateral upper motor neuron leg weakness. The ipsilateral arm is held flexed and adducted while the ipsilateral leg is extended (pyramidal pattern of weakness). To move the affected leg, patients tilt their pelvis to be able to swing the affected leg forward in a 'circumduction' manner.

Spastic gait

Spastic gait is caused by bilateral upper motor neuron leg weakness. Both legs are spastic and patients walk in small steps with their toes pressing firmly on the

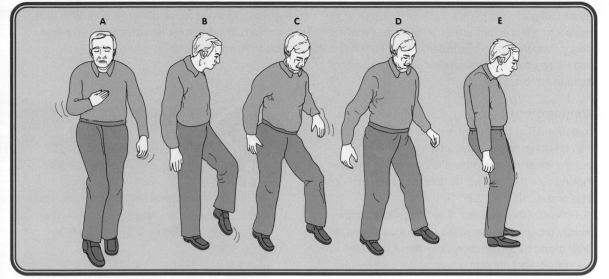

Fig. 12.7 Gait disorders. (A) Hemiplegic, (B) unilateral footdrop, (C) sensory ataxia, (D) cerebellar ataxia, and (E) parkinsonian.

floor as if they are walking in mud. The legs are held in adduction with the knees touching each other, giving the gait a 'scissored' quality.

Cerebellar ataxic gait
Cerebellar ataxic gait (Fig. 12.7D) is caused by cerebellar (and occasionally vestibular) lesions. Patients walk on a wide base and appear unsteady, with erratic body movements. They stagger to the affected side in unilateral lesions (backwards if the lesion is in the cerebellar vermis). Mild cases can be detected only by asking patients to walk on a narrow base (heel–toe walking).

Sensory ataxic gait
Sensory ataxic gait (Fig. 12.7C) is caused by proprioceptive sensory loss. The gait is rather unsteady but patients are able to compensate to some extent using their visual input. Patients tend to stamp their feet down against the floor, owing to the loss of all sensory input, giving the gait a 'stamping' quality. Patients become very ataxic in the dark or if the eyes are closed (see Romberg's test, p. 144).

Footdrop gait
Footdrop gait (Fig. 12.7B) is caused by common peroneal nerve lesion (if unilateral), or peripheral neuropathy (if bilateral). Patients over-flex the hip and the knee to be able to lift their toes off the floor, giving the gait a high-stepping quality.

Parkinsonian gait
Parkinsonian gait (Fig. 12.7E) is caused by Parkinson's disease. Gait is slow and shuffling with small stride length, flexed posture, and reduced arm swinging. Patients often have problems in starting to walk and in turning while walking which is achieved by using an exaggerated number of steps. This gait should be differentiated from the less common *marche à la petit pas* seen in bilateral frontal lobe lesions, in which gait is shuffling but the arms and the trunk are not affected.

Waddling gait
Waddling gait is caused by proximal myopathy. Patients have exaggerated lumbar lordosis. They bend their pelvis forward and walk with a waddle, tilting from one side to the other.

Antalgic gait
Antalgic gait is caused by painful musculoskeletal conditions. Patients walk with a 'limp' in an attempt to minimize the use of the painful leg.

Apraxic gait
Apraxic gait is caused by parietal lobe lesions. Patients have no difficulty in manipulating their limbs when sitting or lying, but when attempting to walk they experience great difficulty in organizing their gait and placing their feet in the right positions. Gait appears to have an odd and bizarre character. Patients are liable to 'freeze' to the ground, unable to initiate movements.

Hysterical gait

Hysterical gait is erratic and unpredictable. Patients stagger widely with exaggerated arm movements. Falls and injuries are unusual but their presence does not exclude this diagnosis.

Romberg's test

To perform Romberg's rest, ask the patient to stand with his or her feet together and assess his or her stability. Next, ask the patient to close his or her eyes, making sure that you will be able to support him or her if he or she falls (Fig. 12.8).

Patients with cerebellar or vestibular lesions are usually ataxic on a narrow base with their eyes open. Their ataxia might get marginally worse when the eyes are closed. Patients with proprioceptive sensory loss might be slightly ataxic on a narrow base with their eyes open, but they fall when they close their eyes (positive Romberg's test).

- Summarize the different types of gait abnormalities.
- State the differences between sensory and cerebellar ataxia, and describe the significance of Romberg's test.

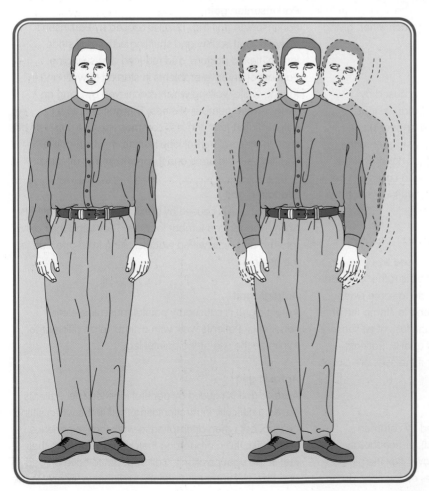

Fig. 12.8 Positive Romberg's test. The patient's stability, satisfactory with the eyes open, immediately deteriorates with the eyes closed.

THE CRANIAL NERVES

Introduction

Examination of cranial nerves plays an important part in an the central nervous system assessment. They provide enormous number of neurological signs that aid localization, particularly in unconscious patients.

Olfactory nerve (I)

To test the olfactory nerves, first ask patients about any recent change in their sense of smell (anosmia, parosmia, olfactory hallucination) (Fig. 12.9). Then, test their ability to smell coffee, cinnamon, and tobacco, by examining each nostril in turn. Avoid using very irritating odours (e.g. ammonia or camphor), which could stimulate the trigeminal nerve endings, even in anosmic patients.

Unilateral loss of smell is usually asymptomatic. Bilateral loss of smell is usually associated with an altered sense of taste (loss of the ability to appreciate aromas).

Remember to examine the olfactory nerve in all patients presenting with personality changes, disinhibition, or dementia (frontal lobe tumours), and in all cases of head injury.

The eye (II and III)
Visual acuity (VA)

Visual acuity is tested using a Snellen chart in a well-lit room. Seat or stand the patient 6 m from the chart. Small, hand-held Snellen charts can be read at a distance of 2 m.

Near visual acuity is tested using reading charts, but this does not necessarily correlate well with distance acuity.

Correct the patient's refractive errors with glasses or a pinhole. Ask the patient to cover each eye in turn with his or her palm, and find which line of print he or she can read comfortably. Visual acuity is expressed as the ratio of the distance between the patient and the chart to the number of the smallest visible line on the chart (normally 6/6) (Fig. 12.10).

If the patient is unable to read characters of line 60 (visual acuity less than 6/60), assess his or her ability to count your fingers at 1m (VA:CF), see your hand movements (VA:HM), or perceive a torch light (VA:LP). If unable to perceive light (VA:NLP), then the patient is medically blind.

Causes of olfactory symptoms

Anosmia (loss of smell)
congenital
nasal sinuses infections/tumours
head injury/cranial surgery
frontal lobe tumours
subfrontal meningiomas
Parosmia (persistent unpleasant smell)
nasal infections/tumours
head injury
depression
Olfactory hallucination
temporal lobe epileptic seizures
Paroxysmal, unpleasant smell (burning rubber, smell of gas)
psychosis

Fig. 12.9 Causes of olfactory symptoms.

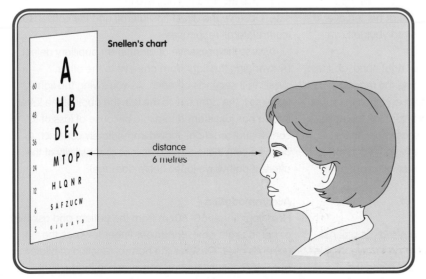

Fig. 12.10 Visual acuity. The patient is able to read line number 24, but not number 12. Visual acuity is 6/24.

Colour vision

Colour vision is tested using Ishahara plates in a daylight-lit room. Test each eye separately. If 13/15 plates or more are read correctly, colour vision can be regarded as normal. This test is designed principally to detect congenital colour vision defects, but is sensitive in detecting mild degrees of optic nerve dysfunction.

Visual fields

Sit about 1m from the patient with your eyes at the same horizontal level. Start by testing for visual inattention. Ask the patient to look into your eyes and hold your hands halfway between you and the patient. Stimulate the patient's visual fields by moving each hand separately and then both hands together, and ask the patient to indicate which of your hands has moved each time.

In patients with parietal lobe lesions, a visual stimulus presented in isolation to the contralateral field is perceived, but it is missed when a comparable stimulus is presented simultaneously to the ipsilateral field.

Visual fields are examined by confrontation, during which you compare your own visual fields with the patient's (provided that yours are normal). The patient's visual field will match yours only if your head positions are exactly comparable and if your hand is exactly halfway between you and the patient; this is seldom the case.

Visual fields in poorly cooperative patients are assessed by using visual threat (sudden, unexpected hand movement into the patient's visual field).

Peripheral fields

Examine each eye in turn. To test the patient's right visual field, ask him or her to cover his or her left eye with his or her left palm and to look into your left eye throughout the examination.

Cover your own right eye with your right hand, and test the patient's peripheral field by bringing the moving fingers of your left hand into the upper and then the lower quadrants of the patient's temporal fields. Ask the patient to inform you as soon as he or she sees your fingers.

Now cover your own right eye with your left hand and examine the patient's nasal fields with your right hand using the same method.

Blind spot

The blind spot is tested using a 10mm red hat pin. Ask the patient to cover his or her left eye and move the pin from the central into the temporal field along the horizontal meridian, having explained to him or her that the pin will disappear briefly and then reappear again, and that he or she should indicate when this happens. Once you have found the patient's blind spot you can map its shape and compare its size with yours.

Central field

The central field is tested by moving a red hat pin along the central visual field (fixation area) in the horizontal meridian. Ask the patient to indicate if the pin disappears (absolute central scotoma) or if the colour appears diminished (relative scotoma). A central scotoma extends temporally from the fixation area into the blind spot.

Visual field defects

Bedside testing of visual fields can detect only large scotomas. Different patterns of visual field defects can be recognized clinically (Fig. 12.11).

Eyelids and pupils

Inspection

Note the position of the eyelids. If there is a ptosis, decide whether it is partial or complete; assess its fatiguability by asking the patient to sustain upward gaze for at least 1 minute. Next, assess the size and shape of the pupils. They should be circular and symmetrical (Fig. 12.12).

Light response

Light responses should be assessed using a bright torch light. Ask the patient to fixate on a distant target and shine the light in each eye in turn from the lateral side. Observe the direct (ipsilateral) and the consensual (contralateral) responses.

Assess the presence of an afferent pupillary defect by swinging the light from one eye to the other, dwelling 3 seconds on each. As you swing the light from, say, the right eye to the left, the pupil of the latter (which has just started to dilate because of loss of its consensual reaction) should immediately constrict. A delayed constriction indicates loss of sensitivity of the afferent pathways (optic nerve damage).

Accommodation

Hold your finger 50–60cm from the patient and ask him or her to fixate on it. Bring your finger towards the patient's eyes. Observe the normal reaction of bilateral pupillary constriction and convergence (adduction).

Fundoscopy

Ask the patient to fixate on a distant target, avoiding bright lights. Using a direct ophthalmoscope, examine the patient's right eye using your right eye, and the patient's left eye using your left eye.

Adjust the ophthalmoscope lens until the retinal vessels are in focus and trace them back to the optic disc. Assess the optic disc shape, colour, and clarity of its margins. The temporal disc margins are normally slightly paler than the nasal margins. The physiological cupping varies in size but does not extend to the disc margins.

Next, assess the retinal vessels. The arteries are narrower than the veins and brighter in colour. The vessels should not be obscured as they cross the disc margins. Look for retinal vein pulsation, which is present in about 80% of normal individuals and is an index of normal intracranial pressure. This is seen best at the disc margins where the veins cross over the arteries. Note the width of the blood vessels and look for arteriovenous nipping at the crossover points.

Assess the rest of the retina, noting any evidence of discoloration, haemorrhages, or white patches of exudate. Ask the patient to look at the light of the ophthalmoscope, which brings the macula into view. Classify fundoscopic abnormalities into those affecting the optic disc, retinal vessels, or the retina (Fig. 12.13).

Patients with acute optic neuritis might have fundoscopic abnormalities similar to papilloedema. However, in the former case, eye movements can be painful and visual acuity is substantially reduced.

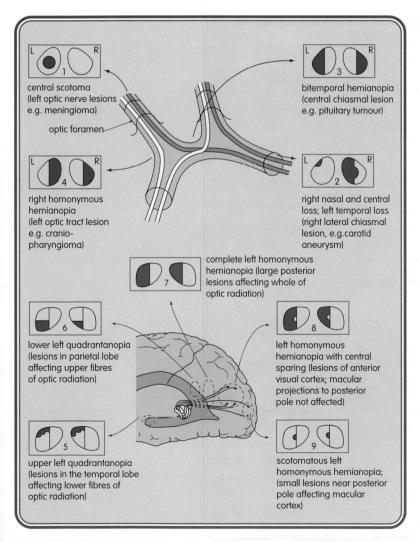

Fig. 12.11 Visual field defects. (Courtesy of Dr Ross, St Thomas's Hospital, London.)

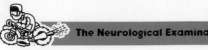
Fig. 12.12 Pupillary abnormalities.

unilateral			reaction to light	associated signs
third nerve palsy			negative	ptosis (partial or complete) external ophthalmoplegia
Horner's syndrome			poor reaction to shade	ptosis (always partial) anhydrosis endophthalmus
Holmes–Adie syndrome			slow reaction	constriction to pilocarpine (0.1%) lower limb areflexia
bilateral				
Argyll Robertson			negative	depigmented iris normal accommodation neurosyphilis
midbrain compression			negative	coma lateralizing signs
pontine stroke			negative	coma hyperventilation hyperpyrexia

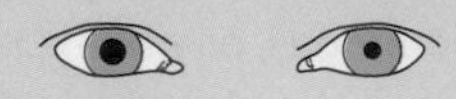

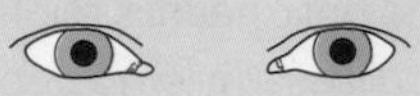

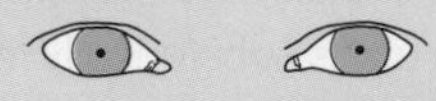

Fig. 12.13 Common fundoscopic abnormalities.

Common fundoscopic abnormalities		
Structure	**Abnormality**	**Pathology**
optic disc	papilloedema	raised intracranial pressure, venous obstruction (e.g. cavernous sinus thrombosis, orbital tumour), high CSF protein (e.g. Guillain–Barré syndrome, spinal cord tumours), malignant hypertension, hypercapnia
	optic atrophy	optic neuritis (e.g. multiple sclerosis, Devic's disease), optic nerve/chiasmal compression (e.g. meningioma, optic nerve gliomas, pituitary tumours, Paget's disease of the skull, arachnoiditis), toxic/metabolic (e.g. methyl alcohol, B_{12} deficiency), long-standing raised intracranial pressure), infections (e.g. neurosyphilis), hereditary (e.g. Leber's optic atrophy)
retinal arteries	silver-wiring, increased tortuosity, arteriovenous nipping	hypertension
	gross narrowing with retinal pallor and reddened fovea	central retinal artery occlusion
	cholesterol or platelet emboli	cerebrovascular disease
retinal veins	venous engorgement	papilloedema (see above), central retinal vein occlusion
retina	haemorrhages	superficial flamed-shaped and deep dot-shaped (hypertension, diabetes) subhyaloid between the retina and the vitreous (subarachnoid haemorrhage)
	exudates	soft cotton-wool and hard exudates (hypertension and diabetes)
	pigmentation	retinitis pigmentosa (e.g. hereditary, Refsum's disease, Kearns–Sayre syndrome), choroidoretinitis (e.g. toxoplasmosis, sarcoidosis, syphilis), post-laser treatment (diabetes)

Eye movements (III, IV, and VI)

Inspect the eyes and note the position of the eyelids and the presence of any strabismus. Strabismus is concomitant (usually asymptomatic) if it remains constant throughout the range of eye movements, and incomitant (paralytic) if it varies.

If the patient is capable of voluntary eye movements, the pursuit and saccadic systems should be tested to assess whether eye movements are conjugate, and to detect the presence of diplopia and nystagmus.

Isolated painful third nerve palsy is suggestive of a posterior communicating artery aneurysm.

Pupil-sparing third nerve palsy is suggestive of vascular aetiology, particularly diabetes.

Monocular diplopia is suggestive of either refractive defects (cornea or lens) or hysteria.

Very complicated and variable diplopia is suggestive of myasthenia gravis. Look for orbicularis oculi weakness in these cases.

Pursuit eye movements

Steady the patient's head with one hand and hold the index finger of your other hand 40–50 cm in front of his or her eyes. Ask the patient to follow your slowly moving finger throughout the range of binocular vision in both the horizontal and the vertical planes in a letter 'H' pattern.

Assess the smoothness, speed, and magnitude of the movements. Look for nystagmus, and ask the patient to report any diplopia. In the presence of diplopia, identify the direction of the maximum separation of images and the two muscles responsible for moving the eyes in this direction (Fig. 12.14). Identify the source of the outer image, which comes from the defective eye, by covering each eye in turn. This will allow you to name the muscle(s) and the nerve(s) involved.

Saccadic eye movements

Ask the patient to keep his or her head still, and to look left, right, up, and down as quickly as possible. Assess the velocity and the accuracy of the movements. Look for slow or absent adduction (internuclear ophthalmoplegia) (Fig. 12.15).

If pursuit or saccadic eye movements are absent, oculocephalic reflex (doll's eye movements) will differentiate between supranuclear and nuclear ocular paralysis. Ask the patient to fixate on your eyes while you rotate his or her head in the horizontal and the vertical planes. In supranuclear lesions the reflex is intact, allowing the patient's eyes to remain fixated on yours.

Ocular nerve paresis

Clinical signs of ocular nerve paresis are shown in Figs 12.16 and 12.17. Causes of ocular paresis are shown in Fig. 12.18.

Nystagmus

Nystagmus is an involuntary rhythmic oscillation of the eyes caused by lesions affecting brainstem vertical and horizontal gaze centres and their vestibular and cerebellar connections. It is usually asymptomatic, except for oscillopsia when patients experience movements of their visual fields.

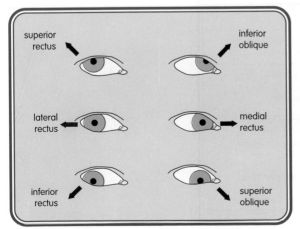

Fig. 12.14 Muscles responsible for eye movements in particular directions.

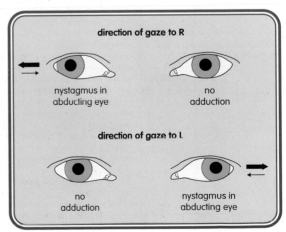

Fig. 12.15 Bilateral internuclear ophthalmoplegia.

Clinical signs of ocular nerve paresis	
Nerve	**Signs**
III	ptosis, eye is deviated laterally and slightly downwards (divergent strabismus), pupil is dilated and not reactive
IV	impaired depression (and intortion) of the fully adducted eye, head might be tilted to the opposite side to avoid diplopia when reading or looking down
VI	impaired abduction (convergent strabismus)

Fig. 12.16 Clinical signs of ocular nerve paresis.

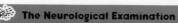

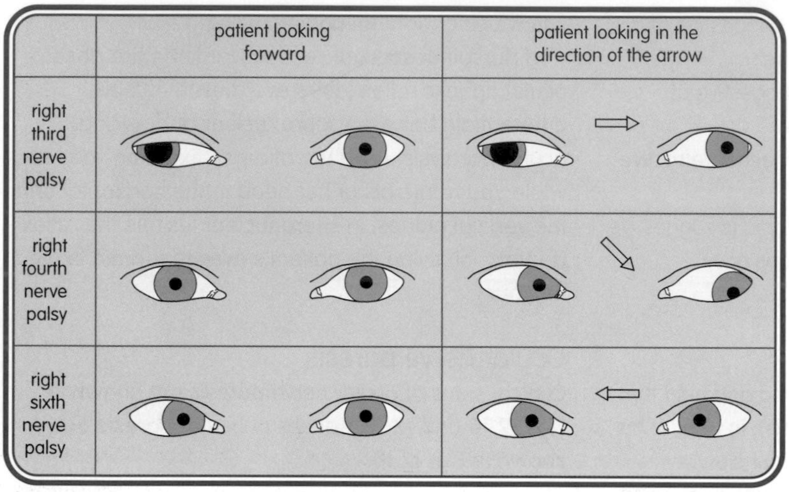

Fig. 12.17 Clinical signs of cranial nerve III, IV, and VI palsies.

Fig. 12.18 Causes of ocular paresis.

Causes of ocular paresis		
Type		**Pathology**
supranuclear gaze paresis	horizontal	frontal lobe lesions: eyes deviated to the side of the lesion pontine lesions: eyes deviated to the opposite side
	vertical	brainstem pretectal region: Parinaud's syndrome (vertical gaze paralysis, pupillary dilation, absent accommodation reflex) extrapyramidal diseases (e.g. Parkinson's disease, progressive supranuclear palsy): impaired vertical gaze (initially upward)
nuclear and nerve (III, IV, VI) palsies	brainstem	vascular lesions, tumours, demyelination, Wernicke's encephalitis
	peripheral	raised intracranial pressure (VI as a false localizing sign, III caused by tentorial herniation) vascular lesions (e.g. atheroma, diabetes, temporal arteritis, syphilis) aneurysms (posterior communicating artery: III; cavernous sinus: III, IV, VI) meningeal inflammation and malignant infiltration skull base tumours (nasopharyngeal carcinoma, chordoma) cranial polyneuropathy (Guillain–Barré syndrome, sarcoidosis) orbital tumours and granulomas, sinus disease
muscle disease		myasthenia gravis, thyroid eye disease, mitochondrial cytopathy

Nystagmus must be differentiated from end-point nystagmoid jerks seen at extreme deviation of gaze, and from the voluntary rapid oscillation of eyes. Both are brief and unsustained.

Testing

Note the presence of nystagmus in the primary position of gaze (when looking forward), and while examining eye movements, and decide whether it is pendular or jerky, and whether the movements are horizontal, vertical, rotatory, or of mixed nature.

Record its amplitude (fine, medium, coarse), persistence, and the direction of gaze in which it occurs (the direction of nystagmus is, by convention, the direction of the fast component). Causes of nystagmus are shown in Fig. 12.19

The face (V and VII)

Trigeminal nerve (V)

Sensory

Sensory testing is performed using the same techniques described later (pp. 164–165). Test light touch, pin prick, and temperature over the forehead, the medial aspects of the cheeks, and the chin, which correspond to the ophthalmic, maxillary, and mandibular branches of the trigeminal nerve, respectively (Fig. 12.20). A partial loss can be detected by comparing the response to the same stimulus on the other sites on the face.

Corneal response is elicited by lightly touching the cornea (not the conjunctiva) with a wisp of cotton wool. Synchronous blinking of both eyes occurs. An afferent defect (Vth cranial nerve lesion) results in depression or absence of the direct and consensual reflex. An efferent defect (VIIth cranial nerve lesion) results in an impairment or absence of the reflex on the side of the facial weakness. The clinical pattern of sensory loss depends on the anatomical site of the lesion (Fig. 12.21).

Motor

Inspect for wasting of the temporalis muscles, which produces hollowing above the zygoma. Ask the patient to clench his or her teeth together and palpate the masseters, noting any wasting. The pterygoid muscles are assessed by resisting the patient's attempts to open his or her mouth. In unilateral trigeminal lesions, the lower jaw deviates to the paralytic side as the mouth is opened.

Jaw jerk

Jaw jerk is a brainstem stretch reflex. Ask the patient to open his or her mouth slightly. Rest your index finger on the apex of the jaw and tap it with the patella hammer. The response, mouth opening, is due to a contraction of the pterygoid muscles. An absent reflex is not significant, but the reflex could be brisk in pseudobulbar palsy (see later).

Fig. 12.19 Causes of nystagmus.

Causes of nystagmus		
Type	**Description**	**Pathology**
pendular	oscillations of equal velocity	long-standing impaired macular vision (since early childhood), miner's nystagmus
jerky	fast phase towards the side of the lesion	unilateral cerebellar lesions
	fast phase to the opposite side of the lesion	unilateral vestibular lesions
	direction of nystagmus varies with the direction of gaze	brainstem pathology
	upbeat nystagmus	lesions at or around the superior colliculi
	downbeat nystagmus	lesions at or around the foramen magnum
rotatory	specific to one head position, and fatigues with repeated testing	unilateral labyrinthine pathology
rotatory or mixed	all other types	brainstem pathology

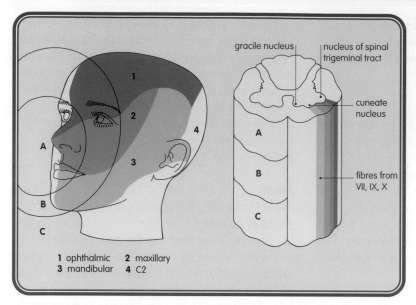

Fig. 12.20 Suggested organization of concentric segments of facial cutaneous innervation within the spinal tract.

1 ophthalmic   2 maxillary
3 mandibular   4 C2

Fig. 12.21 Clinical syndromes of the trigeminal nerve.

Clinical syndromes of the trigeminal nerve		
Site of lesion	**Signs**	**Pathology**
dorsal pons	altered light touch, with preserved pain and temperature.	vascular, tumour
high central medulla	'onion-skin' circumoral analgesia which advances outwards	syringobulbia
low central medulla or high intrinsic cervical lesion above C2	'onion-skin' analgesia which starts at the peripheral parts of the face and advances towards the nose and the mouth	syringomyelia
lateral medulla	ipsilateral loss of pain and temperature	lateral medullary syndrome
upper cervical cord, foramen magnum	generalized sensory loss which starts first in ophthalmic division and advances downwards	cervical spondylosis, meningiomas
sensory root or ganglia	generalized sensory loss of all modalities	acoustic neuroma, meningioma, angioma
peripheral branch	selective sensory loss of all modalities	orbital tumours, neuromas

Facial nerve (VII)

Motor response

Inspect the patient's face, looking for asymmetry of the nasolabial folds and the position of the two angles of the mouth. Assess the movements of the upper part of the face by asking the patient to elevate his or her eyebrows, close his or her eyes tightly, and resist your attempt to open them. Movements of the lower side of the face are assessed by asking the patient to blow out his or her cheeks with air, purse his or her lips tightly together and resist your attempt to open them, show his or her teeth, or whistle. Finally, ask the patient to smile, and observe for any facial asymmetry.

If you detect any weakness or asymmetry, decide if the weakness is confined to the lower part of the face (upper motor neuron lesion) or both the upper and the lower parts of the face (lower motor neuron lesion) (Figs 12.22 and 12.23).

Clinical syndromes of facial weakness		
Site of lesion	**Signs**	**Common pathology**
supranuclear	contralateral (or ipsilateral) UMN weakness	vascular, tumour
brainstem	ipsilateral LMN weakness	vascular, tumours, syrinx, demyelination
cerebellopontine angle	Ipsilateral LMN weakness	acoustic neuromas, meningiomas, angioma
basal meninges	often bilateral LMN weakness	sarcoidosis, malignant meningitis
petrous bone	ipsilateral LMN weakness	middle ear infections, Bell's palsy, geniculate herpetic zoster
face	ipsilateral LMN weakness	parotid tumours, trauma
muscle disease	usually bilateral LMN weakness	myasthenia gravis, myotonic dystrophy, muscular dystrophy
others	usually bilateral LMN weakness	Guillain–Barré syndrome

Fig. 12.22 Clinical syndromes of facial weakness. (LMN, lower motor neuron; UMN, upper motor neuron.)

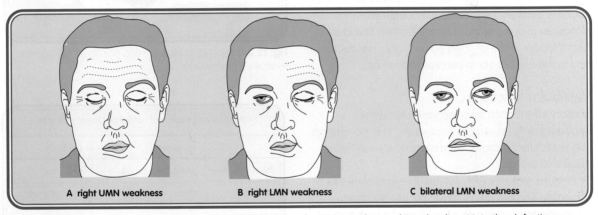

A right UMN weakness   B right LMN weakness   C bilateral LMN weakness

Fig. 12.23 Facial weakness. The patient is asked to close his or her eyes and purse his or her lips. Note the defective eye closure and Bell's phenomenon in B and C. (LMN, lower motor neuron; UMN, upper motor neuron.)

Do not miss bilateral facial weakness. In this case, the face appears to sag, with lack of facial expression.

Look for Bell's phenomenon (eyeball rotates upwards and outwards on attempting to close the eye). The lack of this sign indicates that the patient is not attempting to close his or her eye (? malingerer).

Taste

Formal assessment of taste is rarely of practical benefit. Taste is examined by applying a solution of salt, sweet (sugar), or sour (vinegar) to the anterior two-thirds of the tongue and comparing the response on the two sides. The mouth should be rinsed with water between testing. Cranial nerve VIII lesions proximal to the middle ear will cause loss of taste.

Hyperacusis

Hyperacusis (undue sensitivity to noise) is suggestive of a lesion proximal to the middle ear, affecting the nerve to the stapedius.

Auditory nerve (VIII)
Hearing

Clinical bedside assessment of hearing is not sensitive, and can detect only gross hearing loss. Audiometry is usually required for detailed assessment. Assess each ear separately while masking the hearing in the other ear by occluding the external meatus with your index finger. Test the patient's hearing sensitivity by whispering numbers into his or her ear and asking him or her to repeat them.

If hearing is impaired, examine the external auditory meatus and the tympanic membrane with an auroscope to exclude infections or wax. Determine if the hearing loss is conductive (middle ear pathology) or perceptive (inner ear pathology) by performing Rinné and Weber's tests.

Rinné test

Place a vibrating 512 Hz tuning fork on the mastoid process (bone conduction) and then hold it close to the ear (air conduction). Ask the patient to determine which sound is loudest. Normally, air conduction is louder than bone conduction (positive Rinné). This discrepancy remains in perceptive deafness, but is reversed in conductive deafness.

Weber's test

Place a vibrating 512 Hz tuning fork at the midline over the vertex and ask the patient to determine whether the sound is perceived equally loudly in both ears (normal status), or in one ear more than the other. Sound is heard louder in the affected ear in conductive deafness, and in the normal ear in perceptive deafness.

Vestibular functions

Sensory information from the vestibular system is important in the control of posture and eye movements. The vestibular functions are assessed by examining these two areas:

- Posture: patients with vestibular lesions complain of vertigo and are mildly ataxic but usually able to compensate, using their visual input. However, patients with acute vestibular lesions can be markedly ataxic, with a tendency to fall towards the affected side.
- Nystagmus: unilateral vestibular dysfunction causes jerky/rotatory nystagmus with the fast phase towards the unaffected side (see nystagmus).

Hallpike's manoeuvre

Hallpike's manoeuvre should be performed in all patients with positional vertigo (vertigo precipitated by a particular head position).

Sit the patient at the side of a couch facing away from the edge. Pull the patient quickly backwards and to one side so that the head hangs about 30–45° below the horizontal plane rotated to one side (Fig. 12.24). Ask the patient to keep his or her eyes open and to report any vertigo, and look for nystagmus. Sit the patient up

and observe any nystagmus. Repeat the manoeuvre to the other side.

If positive, repeat the manoeuvre to the same side and determine if the pathology is central or peripheral (not always easy) (Fig. 12.25).

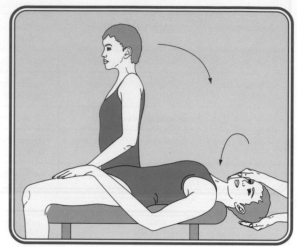

Fig. 12.24 Technique for exhibiting positional nystagmus (Hallpike's manoeuvre).

Features of peripheral and central positional nystagmus		
	Peripheral	**Central**
site of pathology	semicircular canals	brainstem
vertigo	always present	may be absent
nystagmus	rotatory	horizontal/rotatory
onset	delayed by 3–10 seconds	immediate
repeated testing	response fatigues	usually does not fatigue

Fig. 12.25 Features of peripheral and central positional nystagmus.

Caloric testing

Establish that the patient's tympanic membranes are intact. With the patient lying supine with the head elevated at 30°, flush 250 mL of cold water (30°C) into the external auditory meatus. After a delay of 20 seconds, this produces a tonic deviation of the eyes to the same side with compensatory nystagmus to the opposite side lasting for more than 1 minute. Unconscious patients with intact vestibular function will have the tonic deviation only.

The test is repeated 5 minutes later with hot water (44°C), which induces tonic deviation of the eyes to the opposite side and compensatory nystagmus to the side of the irrigated ear.

Labyrinthine or vestibular nerve lesions cause depression of both the 'hot' and the 'cold' responses from the affected side (canal paresis), whereas central lesions cause an enhancement of nystagmus in one of the directions, whether triggered by hot or cold water (directional preponderance).

Clinical patterns of cranial nerve VIII lesions are shown in Fig. 12.26.

The mouth (IX, X, and XII)
Mouth and tongue
Inspect the tongue as it lies in the floor of the mouth for evidence of wasting (unilateral or bilateral), fasciculations (shimmering movements at the surface of the tongue), or other involuntary movements (Huntington's chorea, orofacial dyskinesia). Ask the patient to protrude his or her tongue, and then, move it rapidly from side to side.

Abnormalities can be caused by unilateral or bilateral upper motor neuron or lower motor neuron lesions (Fig. 12.27).

Pharynx and gag reflex
With the patient's mouth wide open, inspect the soft palate, the uvula, and the posterior pharyngeal wall at rest and during phonation (by asking the patient to say 'aah'). Press the end of an orange stick into the posterior pharyngeal wall, first on one side then the other. Assess the afferent pathway of the gag reflex (IXth cranial nerve) by asking the patient if the sensation is comparable on the two sides, and the efferent pathway (Xth cranial nerve) by inspecting the normal response of a symmetrical rise of the soft palate in the midline.

The upper motor neuron innervation of the palatal and pharyngeal muscles is bilateral, and unilateral lesions cause no significant dysfunction. In unilateral lower motor neuron lesions, the palate lies slightly lower on the affected side and deviates to the intact side during phonation or while testing the gag reflex.

Minor and inconsistent deviations of the uvula should be ignored.

The larynx
Formal assessment of the vocal cords is usually done by indirect laryngoscopy, which is not part of the clinical examination. Bedside evaluation is confined to the assessment of phonation and cough.

Clinical patterns of VIIIth nerve lesions		
Site of lesion	**Clinical features**	**Pathology**
peripheral	auditory and/or vestibular symptomatology	cranial trauma barotrauma infections occlusion of the internal auditory artery Ménière's disease toxins and drugs
central	auditory or vestibular symptomatology, often with other cranial nerve involvement (V, VII) and long tract signs	cerebrovascular disease multiple sclerosis cerebellopontine angle tumours brainstem tumours syringobulbia

Fig. 12.26 Clinical patterns of VIIIth cranial nerve lesions.

Clinical patterns of tongue weakness		
lower motor neuron lesions	unilateral	focal atrophy, fasciculations, and deviation to the ipsilateral (paralysed) side
	bilateral	see bulbar palsy (Fig. 12.28)
upper motor neuron lesions	unilateral	deviation to the paralysed side
	bilateral	see pseudobulbar palsy (Fig. 12.28)

Fig. 12.27 Clinical patterns of tongue weakness.

Unilateral lesions of the recurrent laryngeal nerve cause partial upper way obstruction with stridor, hoarseness of voice, and 'bovine' cough. Bilateral lesions cause severe stridor and aphonia.

The accessory nerve (XI)

The function of the trapezius muscles is assessed by asking the patient to elevate his or her shoulders, first without, and then against, resistance. The bulk and the strength of the sternocleidomastoid muscle is assessed by asking the patient to rotate his or her head to the contralateral side against the resistance of your hand.

Bulbar and pseudobulbar palsies (IX, X, XII)

These syndromes describe bilateral weakness of the bulbar muscles of either an upper or a lower motor neuron type (Fig. 12.28).

Multiple cranial nerve palsies
Patchy loss of function

These palsies are usually caused by:

- Malignant meningitis (due to carcinoma, lymphoma, or leukaemia).
- Granulomatous meningitis (due to sarcoidosis, tuberculosis, or syphilis).
- Bone disease (due to metastasis or Paget's disease).

Diffuse loss of function

These palsies are usually caused by:

- Guillain–Barré syndrome.
- Motor neuron disease.
- Myasthenia gravis.
- Polymyositis.

Clinical features and causes of pseudobulbar and bulbar palsies			
	Clinical features	**Cause**	**Pathology**
pseudobulbar palsy	dysarthria (spastic), choking attacks, emotional lability; the tongue is stiff, spastic, slow but not wasted; jaw jerk and gag reflexes are brisk	bilateral upper motor neuron lesions (supranuclear)	cerebrovascular disease, motor neuron disease, multiple sclerosis, supranuclear palsy, Creutzfeldt–Jakob disease
bulbar palsy	dysarthria (nasal), dysphagia and nasal regurgitation; the tongue appears, wasted, flaccid, and fasciculating, and the gag reflex is absent	bilateral lower motor neuron lesions	• nuclear: medullary infarction, tumour, syrinx, encephalitis • peripheral nerve: cranial polyneuropathy (e.g. Guillain–Barré syndrome, sarcoidosis, diphtheria), neoplasms (e.g. meningeal infiltration, metastasis), skull base lesions (e.g. metastasis,chordoma, glomus tumour), skull base anomaly (e.g. Chiari malformation) • disorders of neuromuscular transmission: myasthenia gravis • primary muscle disease: polymyositis, muscular dystrophy

Fig. 12.28 Clinical features and causes of pseudobulbar and bulbar palsies.

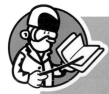

- Explain the significance of olfactory nerve lesions.
- Describe how to examine visual acuity and visual fields. List the most common patterns of field defects.
- Summarize the types of pupillary abnormalities.
- Describe how to examine eye movements. What are the broad differences between the different types of nystagmus?
- Write short notes on the different patterns of trigeminal and facial deficits.
- Describe Rinné and Weber's tests, and Hallpike's manoeuvre.
- What are the differences between pseudobulbar and bulbar palsy?

THE MOTOR SYSTEM

General notes

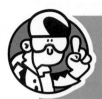

An examination of the motor system should include the following four features. Memorize them.

- Tone
- Power
- Reflexes
- Coordination

In most cases, the cardinal sign of motor impairment is weakness. Remember that other findings (signs) will vary with the sites of pathology (Fig. 12.29).

Acute upper motor neuron lesions cause decreased tone (flaccid paralysis) and absent reflexes, although the Babinski response (see below) will be extensor.

Begin, wherever possible by an inspection of the patient's gait, as outlined on p. 142. In addition, while the patient is standing:

- Can the patient stand on his or her toes and heels without support?
- Can the patient hop? Most patients with significant leg weakness cannot hop.

Following this, ask the patient to lie on the bed, and make sure his or her arms and legs are exposed.

Inspection

When inspecting the patient, look for:

- Wasting—a reduction of muscle bulk in certain muscles compared with others. Wasted muscles are usually weak, and wasting is characteristic of lower motor neuron (i.e. anterior horn cell, nerve root, and nerve) dysfunction.
- Scars—indicating previous injury or surgery, which may have damaged a nerve.
- Fasciculations—seen as rippling or twitching of a muscle at rest, a feature of lower motor neuron problems (especially, but not exclusively, motor neuron disease).
- Involuntary movements such as tremor may be obvious.

Tone

'Tone' means how floppy (decreased tone) or stiff (increased tone) a limb feels. Some patients with increased tone in the legs may complain that their legs 'jump', especially in bed.

Some patients have difficulty relaxing during an examination, which can artificially increase stiffness in their limbs. You must therefore do your utmost to put them at ease.

Arms

To examine tone, relax the patient and ask him or her to make him- or herself 'go floppy'. Take his or her arm and slowly flex and extend the elbow, then hold his or her hand, with the elbow flexed, and pronate/supinate the forearm. If tone is increased you may feel a 'supinator catch'—an interruption of the smooth movement on supination.

Variation in examination findings with site of pathology				
Site of lesion	Wasting	Tone	Power	Reflexes
upper motor neuron	none	increased	decreased	increased
lower motor neuron	wasted	decreased	decreased	decreased
neuromuscular junction	rarely	usually normal, decreased	decreased (fatiguable)	usually normal
muscle	sometimes	normal	decreased	decreased

Fig. 12.29 Variation in examination findings with site of pathology. Not every patient will have every feature and occasionally patients may diverge from these features, but this remains a useful guide.

Legs

There are several ways to examine tone in the legs:

- Rock each leg from side to side on the bed, holding it at the knee. Normally, the foot lags behind the leg. If tone is increased, the foot and leg move stiffly, as one unit. If tone is decreased, the foot flops from side to side.
- Flex and extend the knee, supporting both the upper leg and the foot.
- Place your hand under the patient's knee and quickly lift the knee about 15 cm; normally the foot will stay on the bed; if tone is increased it may jump up with the lower leg.

Clonus describes the rhythmic contractions evoked by a sudden passive stretch of a muscle, elicited most easily at the ankle. A few beats may be normal in anxious patients, but 'sustained clonus' is characteristic of an upper motor neuron lesion.

Increased tone occurs in two main forms:

- Spasticity (derived from the Greek word *spastikos*, to tug or draw) is associated with upper motor neuron lesions, characterized by resistance to the first few degrees of movement, then a sudden lessening of resistance with a 'give way' (so-called clasp-knife) effect.
- Rigidity is characteristic of extrapyramidal disorders such as Parkinson's disease, distinguished clinically from spasticity by constant resistance to passive movement at a joint (lead-pipe rigidity). If tremor is superimposed on rigidity, the resistance is jerky or of 'cog-wheel' type.

Power

Power needs to be tested in each of the main muscle groups. Power in each muscle is given a grade defined

The MRC scale	
Grade	**Response**
0	no movement
1	flicker of muscle when patient tries to move
2	moves, but not against gravity
3	moves against gravity but not against resistance
4	moves against resistance but not to full strength
5	full strength (you cannot overcome the movement)

Fig. 12.30 The MRC scale.

by the Medical Research Council (MRC) scale (Fig. 12.30), which can initially seem complicated, but is very useful for assessing changes.

The scheme in Figs 12.31 and 12.32 allows testing of the main muscle groups of the arms. The scheme in Figs 12.33 and 12.34 allows testing of the main muscle groups of the legs.

Reflexes

Tendon reflexes are most easily determined by briskly stretching the tendon with a tendon hammer, held near the end and briskly tapped either onto the tendon directly or onto a finger placed over the tendon (biceps and supinator) (Fig. 12.35A). You should examine the tendon reflexes shown in Fig. 12.35B. These may be

- Increased.
- Decreased.
- Absent.

If absent, this should be confirmed by reinforcement (Fig. 12.35C). Tendon reflexes are conventionally notated as shown in Fig. 12.36. Abdominal reflexes can be tested as shown in Fig. 12.35D. The plantar response is elicited by scratching of the sole (Fig. 12.35E)

Coordination

Whether a patient can perform smooth and accurate movements is dependent partly on power in the muscles, lack of which may cause clumsiness, but more importantly on the cerebellar system. Assess:

- Gait—a wide-based, sometimes lurching gait is seen in cerebellar disease. Unsteadiness is made more obvious if the patient is asked to walk 'heel to toe'.
- Arms—the finger–nose test: ask the patient to touch your finger, held about 50 cm in front of the patient, with his or her index finger and then to touch his or her nose, then move back and forth. You may have to move the patient's finger for him or her on the first attempt. Cerebellar lesions may cause 'overshooting' of the target, missing your finger (past-pointing), or tremor (intention tremor). Dysdiadochokinesis describes the impairment of rapid alternating movements seen in such patients, and is tested by asking them to slap their palm whilst alternately pronating and supinating their arm.
- Legs—the heel–shin test: ask the patient to place one heel on the other knee, and slowly slide the heel down the lower leg, then up again. Intention tremor may be seen.

Note that the presence of inaccuracy is the most important sign. These movements must be tested on each side in turn.

Abnormality of these movements in a patient with a cerebellar problem is described as ataxia, and may be associated with other signs of cerebellar disease:
- Nystagmus (pp. 149–151).
- Dysarthria (p. 137).

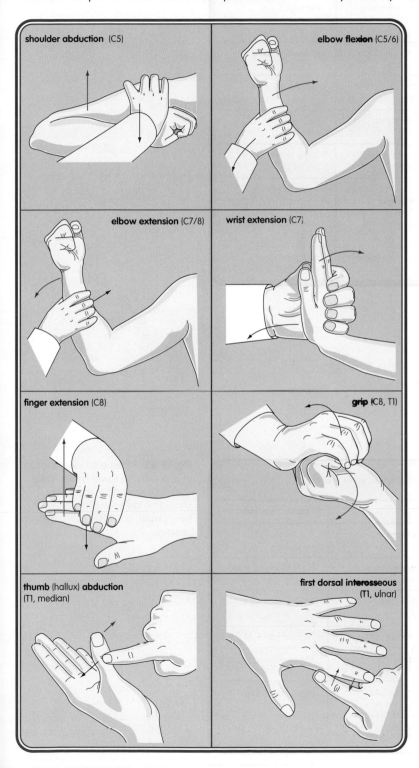

Fig. 12.31 Testing muscle groups of the upper limb. The blue arrow indicates the direction of movement of the patient, and the black arrow the direction of movement of the examiner. Each muscle group should be given a grade as defined by the MRC scale (see Fig. 12.30).

shoulder abduction (C5)

elbow flexion (C5/6)

elbow extension (C7/8)

wrist extension (C7)

finger extension (C8)

grip (C8, T1)

thumb (hallux) abduction (T1, median)

first dorsal interosseous (T1, ulnar)

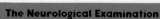
Scheme for examination of power in the upper limbs		
Movement	**Instruction**	**Muscle/myotome**
shoulder abduction	hold your arms out to the side, keep them there and don't let me stop you	deltoid/C5
elbow flexion	bend your elbow and don't let me straighten it	biceps/C5, C6
elbow extension	now straighten your elbow and don't let me bend it	triceps/C7, C8
wrist extension	cock your hands up like this and don't let me stop you	wrist extensors/C7
finger extension	straighten your fingers out and don't let me push them down	finger extensors/C8
grip	grip my fingers	finger flexors/C8, T1
thumb abduction	[with palms flat] Point your thumb to the ceiling and don't let me push it down	abductor pollicis brevis/C8, T1, median nerve
index finger abduction	spread your fingers wide and don't let me push them together	abductors (dorsal interossei)/T1, ulnar nerve

Fig. 12.32 Scheme for examination of power in the upper limbs. It is useful to get into the habit of giving the same instruction to each patient you examine.

Scheme for examination of power in the lower limbs		
Movement	**Instruction**	**Muscle/myotome**
hip flexion	lift your leg straight off the bed, keep it up	iliopsoas/L1, L2
hip adduction	keep your knees together and don't let me pull them apart	hip adductors/L2, L3
knee extension	straighten your knee and don't let me bend your leg	quadriceps/L3, L4
knee flexion	bend your knee and keep it bent	hamstrings/L5, S1
ankle dorsiflexion	pull your foot up towards your nose, don't let me push it down	tibialis anterior and long extensors/L4, L5
plantiflexion (towards the floor)	point your foot down to the bed, keep it there	gastrocnemius/S1
knee extension	press your legs flat against the bed and don't let me pull them up	gluteal muscles/L5, S1

Fig. 12.33 Scheme for examination of power in the lower limbs. Ideally, knee flexion and hip extension should be tested with the patient lying prone, but this is rarely done in practice.

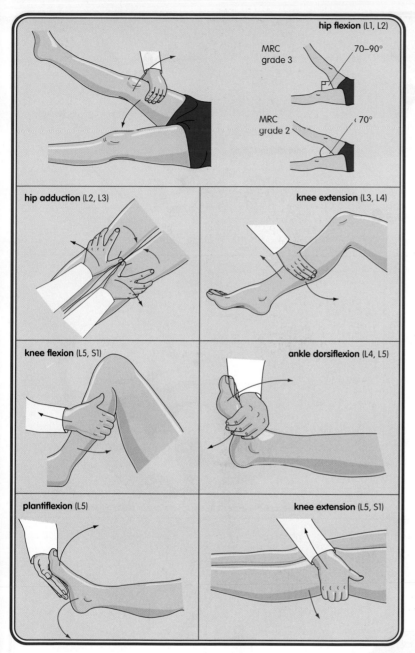

Fig. 12.34 Testing muscle groups of the lower limb. The blue arrow indicates the direction of movement of the patient, and the black arrow the direction of movement of the examiner. Each muscle group should be given a grade as defined by the MRC scale (see Fig. 12.30).

hip flexion (L1, L2)

MRC grade 3   70–90°

MRC grade 2   ‹ 70°

hip adduction (L2, L3)

knee extension (L3, L4)

knee flexion (L5, S1)

ankle dorsiflexion (L4, L5)

plantiflexion (L5)

knee extension (L5, S1)

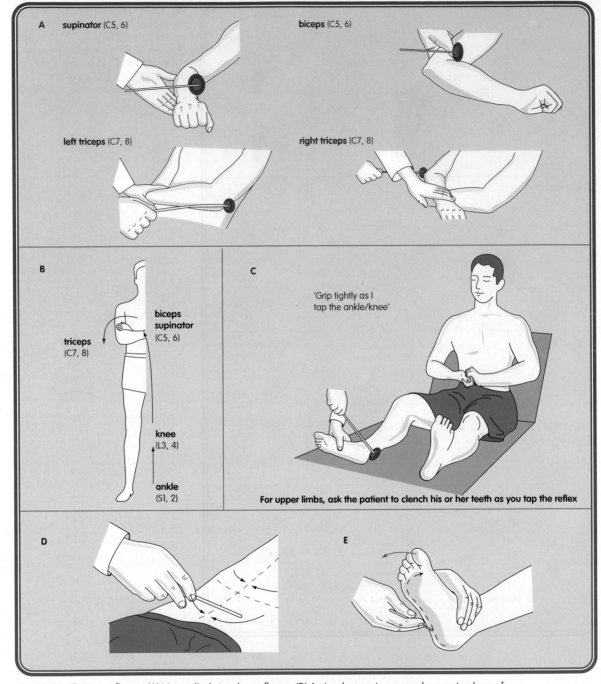

Fig. 12.35 Eliciting reflexes. (A) Upper limb tendon reflexes. (B) A simple way to remember root values of reflexes. (C) Testing ankle jerk with reinforcement. (D) Abdominal reflexes: test in four quadrants shown. (E) The normal response is a downgoing hallux. In an upper motor neuron lesion, the hallux dorsiflexes and the other toes fan out (the Babinski response).

Fine movements

Early stages of an upper motor neuron or extrapyramidal disorder may be picked up by noting impairment of fine finger movements: Ask the patient to pretend to play a piano, and to touch each of his or her fingers in turn with the thumb of the same hand.

Abnormal movements (dyskinesias)

Abnormal movements include:

- Decreased movement, e.g. the bradykinesia of Parkinson's disease.
- Increased movement.

The main types of increased movement you will encounter are shown in Fig. 12.37, and may involve the limbs (more usually the arms) and face. All are involuntary.

Annotation of tendon reflexes	
normal	+
brisk	++
very brisk, with associated clonus	+++
absent	0
present with reinforcement only (decreased)	±

Fig. 12.36 Annotation of tendon reflexes.

Types of abnormal movement (dyskinesia)		
Tremor	**action** physiological	normal, low amplitude, in outstretched hands
	drug induced	exaggeration of normal (e.g. sympathomimetics, lithium)
	essential	coarser, especially when assuming a posture (e.g. holding a glass); usually autosomal dominant; especially in upper limbs; may involve the head (titubation)
	resting	ask the patient to sit with his hands in his lap, most common in Parkinson's disease
	intention	cerebellar, as above
Jerks	**tic**	abrupt, repetitive, stereotyped jerk-like movements; especially facial; no cause is often found; can be suppressed
	chorea	fleeting, irregular, semi-purposeful, disorderly movements affecting any body part; caused by (e.g.) Huntington's disease, stroke involving the subthalamic nucleus (causing ipsilateral chorea, or hemiballismus), drugs (e.g. neuroleptics), or systemic lupus erythematosus
	athetosis	slow, writhing movements, often with chorea
	myoclonus focal segmental generalized	brief, shock-like muscle contractions of 1 body part (e.g. palatal myoclonus) caused by focal disease of the spinal cord or brainstem and involving body segments supplied by this region (e.g. arm) a large number of causes including liver and renal failure, Creutzfeldt–Jakob disease, anoxia, and myoclonic epilepsy May also be *at rest*, with *action* (e.g. postanoxia), or *stimulus sensitive* (e.g. postencephalitis)
Dystonia	**focal segmental axial hemidystonia generalized**	sustained muscle contraction causing unusual postures, may be painful involving one body part (e.g. writers' cramp, torticollis) affecting adjacent body segments involving neck and back on one side of the body (e.g. cerebral palsy) all limbs and axial muscles involved (e.g. metabolic disorders—Wilson's disease, Parkinson's disease) drug-induced dystonia may be acute (e.g. metaclopramide, neuroleptics), or chronic (e.g. L-dopa, phenytoin)

Fig. 12.37 Types of abnormal movement (dyskinesia).

The most important aspect of examination of dyskinesias is inspection, and most of the features described in Fig. 12.37 can be elicited by this alone. In addition:

- Tremor at rest—ask the patient to sit with his or her hands overhanging his or her lap, close his or her eyes and count backwards from 100 to 'bring out' resting tremor.
- Tremor with different actions—the patient will complain if anything in particular makes his or her tremor worse (e.g. holding a cup), so examine those actions in particular. The same applies to myoclonus and dystonias.
- Walking may exaggerate certain movement disorders (e.g. dystonias), so examine this too.

The akinetic rigid syndromes are characterized by abnormal movement:

- Parkinson's disease.
- Steele–Richardson syndrome (with vertical eye movement disturbance and mild dementia).
- Multiple system atrophy (MSA; Chapter 16):
  - Shy–Drager syndrome (with autonomic failure).
  - Striatonigral degeneration (like Parkinson's but often not responsive to treatment).
  - Olivopontocerebellar atrophy.

When examining a patient with Parkinson's disease, the most commonly encountered disorder of movement, look in particular for:

- Festinant gait—slow, shuffling, flexed, decreased arm swing, unstable on turning, may 'freeze'. May show retropulsion (will walk backwards if stopped). Initiation of movements is affected, so watch the patient rise from a chair, or start to walk from a stationary position.
- Bradykinesia (slow movements) especially obvious on fine finger movements, as above.
- Rigidity—carefully examine tone for cog-wheeling.
- Tremor—pill-rolling, at rest.
- Facial akinesia—characteristic facies with poverty of movement and lack of expression. May have a 'positive glabellar tap': with the hand above the patient, repeatedly tap between the eyes. A normal person will stop blinking after a few taps, but a patient with Parkinson's disease will continue to blink. In practice, this is not particularly useful, but is a favourite with examiners. Increased salivation or drooling may also be evident.

- Handwriting—small and cramped. Keep a sample of this in your examination notes.

Causes of mixed upper and lower motor neuron signs:
○ **Motor neuron disease**
○ **Single spinal cord and adjacent root lesion (e.g. cervical spondylosis)**
○ AIDS
○ Syphilis
○ **Chronic upper motor neuron weakness causing 'disuse atrophy'**

○ **What are the important features in examination of the motor system?**
○ **Classify tone, and give examples of each type.**
○ **Describe your assessment of a patient you suspect may have a disorder of coordination.**
○ **Describe your approach towards a patient you think has Parkinson's disease.**

SENSATION

General notes

Patients use various terms to describe sensory disturbance, including numbness, weakness, tingling/pins and needles (paraesthesia), odd unpleasant touch (dysaesthesia), and painful touch (hyperaesthesia).

Tell the patient that you are going to test whether he or she can feel certain sensations. Test each sensation in turn (rather than each limb in turn); it will be easier to remember what you have found and will be quicker to do.

Sensory testing

Do not spend hours doing this, you will exhaust the patient and yourself. Be sensible, and tailor you examination to the patient's complaint.

Remember, sensation from one side of the body travels in sensory tracts to the contralateral cerebral hemisphere.

If the patient complains of loss of sensation, start sensory testing in the abnormal area, and move out from there.

The dermatomes of the upper and lower limbs are shown in Fig. 12.38.

Pin prick

Use a sensory testing/needlework pin, not a needle. With the patient's eyes open, start at the tips of the fingers/toes and work your way proximally. If the patient does not complain of sensory disturbance, it is not necessary to traverse the entire body with the pin. Remember, this is testing *pain* sensation. Ask the patient 'is it sharp or blunt?'

Light touch

Test with cotton wool and with the patient's eyes closed. Start at fingers/toes and work proximally. Ask the patient to 'say yes when you feel me touching you'.

Joint position sense

Move the dorsal interphalangeal (DIP) joint of the index finger/toe up or down, holding the sides of the digit. Ask the patient 'is your toe/finger moving up . . . or down?'

Vibration sense

Use a 128 Hz tuning fork. Set it vibrating, and place it on the patient's sternum. Ask the patient 'can you feel this vibrating?' Place the tuning fork on the DIP joint of the finger or big toe (hallux). Ask 'can you feel it now?'

Sensation is often lost early in neuropathies.

Two-point discrimination

Test two-point discrimination with specific compasses and with the patient's eyes closed. While testing on the pulp of the index finger (normal 3 mm) and hallux (5 mm), ask 'do you feel one point or two?'

Temperature

With the patient's eyes closed, touch the skin with the flat forks of a tuning fork, not vibrating. Ask, 'does this feel hot or cold?'

Lhermitte's symptom

Lhermitte's symptom is a sudden, electric-shock-like sensation travelling down the neck and back when the neck flexes, caused by a lesion in the spinal cord, most typically multiple sclerosis.

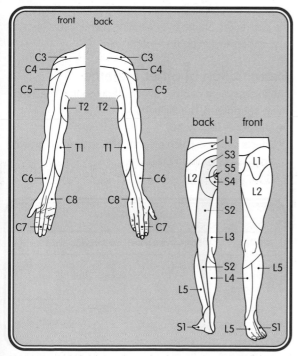

Fig. 12.38 The dermatomes of the upper and lower limbs.

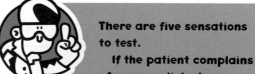

There are five sensations to test.

If the patient complains of sensory disturbance, start testing that area first. If there is no complaint, start distally and move proximally.

Testing each sensation in turn rather than each limb in turn is simplest.

Pain sensation is not agony sensation and therefore do not use a blood-taking needle.

Vibration sense is often lost in neuropathies.

- ○ **Describe the pattern of sensory loss you would expect in a patient with disease affecting the right cervical dorsal column. Give examples of pathology that could cause this.**
- ○ **How would you examine a patient who presented with tingling extremities? What sorts of disease cause such symptoms?**

THE AUTONOMIC NERVOUS SYSTEM

The structure and function of the autonomic nervous system has been outlined in Chapter 6. This, under largely involuntary control, innervates all the viscera, influenced by the hypothalamus via both direct descending pathways and endocrine hormones. It is important to appreciate the anatomy and roles of the individual sympathetic and parasympathetic systems, especially in relation to the effects of drugs on each. However, clinically, 'autonomic failure' usually involves both systems simultaneously, most commonly presenting with a combination of symptoms, as in Fig. 12.39.

Thorough examination of this system is not necessary in every neurological patient unless the patient complains of symptoms of autonomic failure or the diagnosis is suspected. The following tests may then be performed at the bedside (more specialized tests may be performed by an autonomic function laboratory).

Examination of the cardiovascular system

Measure the blood pressure after the patient has been lying down for a few minutes. Then stand the patient up, wait for a minute and take the blood pressure again. The systemic blood pressure normally rises a little. A fall of >20mmHg is abnormal.

The pulse can be monitored by a continuous electrocardiogram recording (measurement of the R–R interval is a useful way of measuring such pulse changes) in response to posture, with deep respiration (sinus arrhythmia may be lost), and with the Valsalva manoeuvre.

The Valsalva manoeuvre

Ask the patient to take a deep breath in, then to blow out through a sphygmomanometer for 12 seconds, maintaining a pressure of 30 mmHg. Normally, a tachycardia occurs during the forced expiration, followed by a reflex bradycardia on release. The blood pressure drops initially, then is maintained throughout the expiration, before overshooting on release. This response is lost in autonomic failure.

Examination of other systems

The examination of other effects of autonomic failure is more specialized, but includes:

- The pupils (Fig. 12.40).
- Effects of stress (such as grip, arousal, mental activity) on pulse and blood pressure.

Signs and symptoms of autonomic failure	
Affected system or site	**Signs and symptoms**
cardiovascular system	postural hypotension (or, uncommonly, hypertension); impaired response of pulse to respiration, posture or Valsalva manouvre; resting tachycardia
genitourinary system	impotence, ejaculatory failure, changes in bladder function (including incontinence)
gastrointestinal tract	constipation or diarrhoea
secretory systems	inability to sweat; dry mouth and eyes
pupils	Horner's syndrome; dilation or constriction; sluggish or absent light response

Fig. 12.39 Signs and symptoms of autonomic failure.

Examination of the pupils		
Test	**Normal response**	**Autonomic failure**
instillation of 1:1000 adrenaline	no effect	dilation if have sympathetic post-ganglionic denervation
instillation of 2.5% methacholine	no effect	constriction if have parasympathetic denervation

Fig. 12.40 Examination of the pupils.

- Pharmacological tests of cardiovascular function.
- Sweating responses with heat and pharmacological agents.
- Skin responses to pharmacological agents.
- Urodynamic tests and sphincter electromyography.

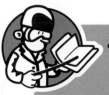

○ **Describe symptoms you would enquire about if suspecting a patient had a disorder of autonomic function.**

○ **How would you go about investigating such symptoms?**

EXAMINATION OF THE UNCONSCIOUS PATIENT

Causes of unconsciousness in adults
See differential diagnosis of coma in Chapter 11 (p. 134).

Assessment of the patient
As with any medical emergency, resuscitation is the priority.

A. Check the airway—in danger either because protective reflexes (e.g. coughing) are suppressed or the respiratory centre is compromised. Clear debris and insert a Guidel airway or endotracheal tube if necessary.

B. Breathing—early stages of respiratory centre depression cause 'periodic' (Cheyne–Stokes) breathing, with alternate hyperventilation and apnoea. Later the patient may hyperventilate. Breathing then becomes irregular, then gasping, prior to respiratory arrest. Give oxygen and count the respiratory rate. Abnormality indicates that artificial ventilation may be necessary.

C. Circulation—pulse and blood pressure. Raised intracranial pressure causes raised blood pressure and a slow pulse, and progression of this indicates increasing pressure. Drug overdoses may cause arrhythmias. Hypotension may need to be corrected. Attach an electrocardiogram monitor.

D. Diabetes—hypoglycaemia is a common and easily treatable cause of unconsciousness (usually caused by insulin overdose); check blood glucose immediately in every unconscious patient, and treat with intravenous dextrose if low. If high, check the urine for ketones and treat diabetic coma.

Assess the patient's general and neurological status (a rapid but careful examination of each system is mandatory). Obtain a history from a relative or friend (this is often the most helpful part of the assessment and can save a great deal of time). Look for drug bottles, prescriptions or a Medic-Alert bracelet.

The Glasgow coma scale (Fig. 12.41) is a widely used, standard, consistent, and fairly sensitive measure of the level of unconsciousness, which enables:

- Small changes in the patient's unconscious level to be noted quickly.
- Medical staff to communicate rapidly with each other regarding the patient's condition.

You should also consider:

- Narcotics (e.g. pin-point pupils, needletracks, slow respiratory rate); give naloxone.
- Is the patient fitting? If so, give intravenous diazepam.
- Head injury (if found, assume also has cervical spine injury until proved otherwise).

Glasgow coma scale		
Eyes (E)		
	opening spontaneously (with blinking)	4
	open to command or speech	3
	open in response to pain (applied to limbs or sternum)	2
	not opening	1
Motor function (M)		
	obeys commands	6
	localizes to pain	5
	withdraws from pain	4
	flexor response to pain (decorticate)	3
	extensor response to pain (decerebrate)	2
	no response to pain	1
Vocalization (V)		
	appropriate speech	5
	confused speech	4
	inappropriate words	3
	groans only	2
	no speech	1

Fig. 12.41 The Glasgow coma scale. Coma score is E+M+V. The maximum (fully conscious) score is therefore 15 and the range 3–15.

- Neck stiffness (e.g. meningitis, subarachnoid haemorrhage). If there is any suspicion of meningitis, do not delay treatment whilst a CT of the brain and lumbar puncture is performed—take blood for culture and treat immediately with intravenous antibiotics.

Particular points to note in the neurological assessment are:

- Pupils, eye movements (Fig. 12.42), and fundi. Papilloedema is a late stage of raised intracranial pressure, and this diagnosis cannot be excluded if the fundi are normal. Retinal haemorrhages may be seen with subarachnoid haemorrhage.
- Tone, power (is there any movement, spontaneously or in response to command or pain?), and reflexes can localize the cause. Brainstem lesions usually cause bilateral (symmetrical or asymmetrical) signs, sometimes just reflex changes. Supratentorial lesions usually cause asymmetrical signs (e.g. hemiparesis).

Investigations

Undertake urgent investigations [e.g. blood glucose, U and Es (urea and electrolytes), LFTs (liver function tests), FBC (full blood count), arterial blood gases, urine and blood drug screens, TFTs (thyroid function tests), blood cultures. CXR (chest X-ray), skull XR, CT brain scan, LP (lumbar puncture), and EEG (electroencephalogram) may also be necessary.

Other management

The patient is likely to need catheterization (also enables fluid balance to be monitored). Other aspects of longer-term care include:

- Continued monitoring of A, B, C, and Glasgow coma scale.
- Turning to prevent pressure sores.
- Eye, mouth, bladder, and bowel care.
- Passive limb movements to prevent contractures.

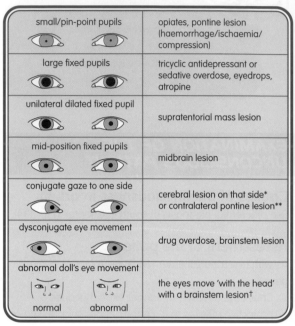

small/pin-point pupils	opiates, pontine lesion (haemorrhage/ischaemia/compression)
large fixed pupils	tricyclic antidepressant or sedative overdose, eyedrops, atropine
unilateral dilated fixed pupil	supratentorial mass lesion
mid-position fixed pupils	midbrain lesion
conjugate gaze to one side	cerebral lesion on that side* or contralateral pontine lesion**
dysconjugate eye movement	drug overdose, brainstem lesion
abnormal doll's eye movement normal abnormal	the eyes move 'with the head' with a brainstem lesion†

Fig. 12.42 Pupils and eye movements in the unconscious patient.* 'looking towards the lesion'; ** 'looking away from the lesion'; †normally, if the head is held and turned quickly from side to side, the eyes swivel in the opposite direction to the head.

An unconscious patient is a medical emergency, and, as such, resuscitation takes priority (A, B, C).

Because hypoglycaemia is easily treatable, a finger-prick glucose test should be done immediately.

The Glasgow coma scale gives an easily recognizable estimation of the level of consciousness.

Pupils, eye movements, tone, and reflexes may be the only source of neurological localization.

- A 21-year-old man is brought to accident and emergency at 3 a.m., having been found unconscious in the street. Describe your management.
- How can changes in a patient's pupils help you understand why they are unconscious?

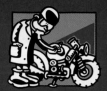

13. Further Investigations

NEUROLOPHYSIOLOGICAL INVESTIGATIONS

Electroencephalography (EEG)

EEG measures electrical potentials generated by the neurons lying underneath an electrode on the scalp, and compares this with either a reference electrode or a neighbouring electrode. The normal trace is symmetrical, and therefore asymmetries, as well as specific abnormalities, may indicate an underlying disorder.

Before accurate brain imaging was possible, EEG was used to detect focal lesions. These are now more commonly picked up with CT or MRI, but EEG remains useful for detecting underlying abnormalities of cerebral function, and especially for:

- Epilepsy (see below).
- Diagnosis of encephalitis.
- In coma.
- Aid to diagnosis of Creutzfeldt–Jakob disease (CJD).
- Diagnosis of subacute sclerosing panencephalitis (SSPE).

The main role of EEG is in the assessment of epilepsy. It can help in the following ways:

- Diagnosis (although the EEG may be normal in patients who have clearly had seizures), with increased yield obtained if recording is made under conditions of sleep deprivation, with hyperventilation, and with photic stimulation.
- Classification of seizure type, which may optimize therapy.
- Assessment for surgical intervention.
- Diagnosis of pseudoseizures (especially with simultaneous video recording—telemetry).

'Invasive EEG monitoring' refers to electrodes inserted directly into the brain, undertaken preoperatively, before surgery to remove an epileptic focus.

Different normal rhythms are characteristically found over different regions of the brain (Figs 13.1 and 13.2). Other than these rhythmic activities, other abnormal activity may be generated in certain conditions (Figs 13.3 and 13.4).

Fig. 13.1 Normal EEG rhythms.

Normal EEG rhythms		
Rhythm	**Characteristics**	**Site and comments**
alpha	8–13 Hz (normal)	posterior; especially with eyes closed
beta	>13 Hz (normal)	anterior; increased with sedatives (e.g. barbiturates)
theta	4–7 Hz (normal)	normal in young and when drowsy
delta	<4 Hz (abnormal except in sleep)	slow rhythm generated over a structural lesion and in sleep

Fig. 13.2 Normal EEG rhythms.

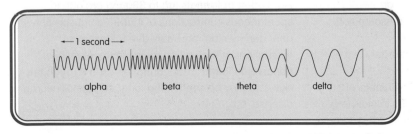

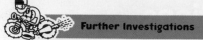

Some abnormal EEG activities	
Activity	**Interpretation**
generalized slow-wave activity	metabolic encephalopathy, drug overdose, encephalitis
focal slow-wave activity	underlying structural lesion
focal/generalized spikes or spike and slow wave activity	epilepsy
three-per-second (3/sec) bilateral, symmetrical spike-and-wave activity (Fig 13.4)	typical absence seizures (idiopathic generalized epilepsy)
periodic complexes (generalized sharp waves every 0.5–2.0 seconds)	CJD

Fig. 13.3 Some abnormal electroencephalographic activities.

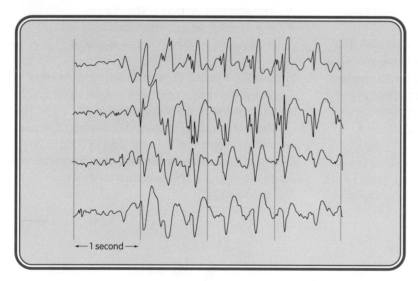

← 1 second →

Fig. 13.4 Three-per-second (3/sec) spike-and-wave activity. Characteristic of typical absence seizure.

Electromyography (EMG) and nerve conduction studies (NCS)

Usually performed together, these investigations examine the integrity of muscle, peripheral nerve, and lower motor neurons. They are useful in:

- Determining the cause of weakness (e.g. neuropathy, myopathy, anterior horn cell disease).
- Determining the distribution of the abnormality (e.g. generalized/focal).
- Suggesting the type of myopathy (e.g. dystrophy or myositis) or neuropathy (e.g. axonal or demyelinating; motor, sensory, or sensorimotor).
- Diagnosing myasthenia gravis.
- Assessing baseline deficits before surgery (e.g. carpal tunnel syndrome).
- Objectively assessing the response to medical therapies, especially new treatments in trials (e.g. human immunoglobulin in Guillain–Barré syndrome).

Normal muscle at rest is electrically silent (apart from actually during needle insertion—insertional activity), unless the needle is placed in the region of a motor end-plate (when miniature end-plate potentials are recorded). During voluntary movement, individual motor unit potentials (MUPs, the activity of a single anterior horn cell) can be seen. Fig. 13.5 shows common abnormalities.

Fibrillations and fasciculations

Fibrillation potentials (up to 300 µV) are due to spontaneous contractions of individual muscle fibres after denervation, probably due to rhythmic fluctuations in the resting membrane potential of denervated fibres. They cannot be seen through the skin, but may be seen in the tongue in motor neuron disease.

Fasciculation potentials (up to 5 mV, usually every 3 or 4 seconds) are contractions of groups of muscle fibres after denervation, visible on both EMG and through the skin as a twitch or ripple. They are especially seen in motor neuron disease. They may be normal , especially in calf muscles, usually at a rate of 1/s.

Other studies

These include:

- Magnetic brain stimulation.
- Evoked potentials (EPs).
  - Visual EPs (VEPs).
  - Brainstem auditory EPs (BSAEPs).
  - Somatosensory EPs (SSEPs).

ROUTINE INVESTIGATIONS

You should be aware of simple tests of neurological relevance. In this section, five areas of investigation are presented:

- Haematology (Fig. 13.6).
- Biochemistry (Fig. 13.7).
- Immunology (Fig. 13.8).
- Microbiology (Fig. 13.9).
- Cerebrospinal fluid findings (Fig. 13.10).

For each test, normal ranges are given, with neurological differential diagnoses for high and low values. Cerebrospinal fluid protein levels are given in g/dL and serum levels are in g/L.

- Describe the uses of the EEG.
- How may EMG and nerve conduction studies aid your understanding of a patient presenting with a weak foot?

Common abnormalities of the EMG and NCS	
Abnormality	**Change in electromyographic trace**
denervation	increased insertional activity; large amplitude, long duration, polyphasic MUPs, fibrillations; fasciculations
myopathy	small, short, polyphasic MUPs
myotonia	high-frequency bursts, sounding like a dive-bomber over a loudspeaker
myasthenia	abnormal decrement on repetitive stimulation; jitter with single-fibre studies (indicating variable neuromuscular transmission time)
Abnormality	**Change in nerve conduction**
axonal neuropathy	small action potential; normal nerve conduction velocity
demyelinating neuropathy	slow nerve conduction velocity; prolonged latency (time to travel from one point to the next); normal or slightly reduced action potential

Fig. 13.5 Common abnormalities found with electromyography (EMG) and nerve conduction studies (NCS). (MUPs, motor unit potenials.)

Haematology			
Test	**Normal range**	**Abnormality**	**Possible interpretation**
full blood count			
haemoglobin (Hb)	13.5–18.0 g/dL male; 11.5–16.0 g/dL female	low; anaemia	may cause non-specific neurological symptoms (e.g. dizziness, weakness, fainting); may suggest an underlying chronic illness
		high; polycythaemia	predisposes to stroke and chorea
mean cell volume (MCV)	76–96 fL	high; macrocytic anaemia	vitamin B_{12} deficiency (peripheral neuropathy, SCDC, dementia)
		low; microcytic anaemia	may indicate an underlying chronic illness; associated with idiopathic intracranial hypertension
white cell count (WBC)			
neutrophils	$2–7.5 \times 10^9$	high; neutrophilia	meningitis or other infection
		low; neutropenia	leukaemia/lymphoma (infiltrative disease, space-occupying lesions, peripheral neuropathy) multiple myeloma (neuropathy, vertebral collapse, hyperviscosity syndrome)
lymphocytes	$1.5–3.5 \times 10^9$	high; lymphocytosis	viral infection (transverse myelitis, Guillain–Barré syndrome)
		low; lymphopenia	leukaemia/lymphoma, as above
eosinophils	$0.04–0.44 \times 10^9$	high; eosinophilia	hypereosinophilic syndrome (rare)
platelet count	$150–400 \times 10^9$	high; thrombocythaemia	predisposes to stroke
		low; thrombocytopenia	intracranial bleeding
erythrocyte sedimentation rate (ESR)	<20 mm/h	high	vasculitis (e.g. PAN, SLE, giant cell arteritis) may cause cerebral, cranial, and peripheral nerve infarcts, confusion and fits)
coagulation tests			
activated partial thromboplastin time (APT or PTTK)	35–45 s	high	SLE; antiphospholipid syndrome
protein C, protein S	varies with laboratory	low; deficiency	inherited predisposition to thrombosis
factor 5 Leiden	varies with laboratory	present	mutation causes a single amino acid substitution in factor 5, which results in activated protein C resistance and predisposition to thrombosis
vitamin B_{12}	>150 ng/L	low; deficiency	peripheral neuropathy, SCDC, confusion/dementia
folate	2.1–2.8 mg/L	low; deficiency	peripheral neuropathy, dementia

Fig. 13.6 Possible consequences of abnormalities in blood or serum levels of haematological indices. Individual laboratories may have different normal ranges.
(APT, activated partial thromboplastin; PAN, polyarteritis nodosa; PTTK, partial thromboplastin time; SCDC, subacute combined degeneration of the cord; SLE, systemic lupus erythematosus.)

Biochemistry			
Test	**Normal range**	**Abnormality**	**Interpretation**
urea and electrolytes (U and Es)			
sodium	135–145 mmol/L	high; hypernatraemia low; hyponatraemia	both may cause weakness, confusion, and fits
potassium	3.5–5.5 mmol/L	high; hyperkalaemia low; hypokalaemia	hyper/hypokalaemic periodic paralysis
urea	2.5–6.7 mmol/L	high; renal failure	confusion, peripheral neuropathy
creatinine	<150 mmol/L	high; renal failure	confusion, peripheral neuropathy
glucose (fasting)	4–6 mmol/L	high; diabetes	neuropathy, coma
		low; hypoglycaemia	confusion, coma, focal signs
calcium	2.2–2.6 mmol/L	low; hypocalcaemia	tetany
liver function tests (LFTs) bilirubin and liver enzymes	bilirubin range: 3–17 μmol/L enzymes vary between laboratories	high	liver disease: confusion, tremor, neuropathy
creatine kinase	24–195 U/L	high	muscle disease: myositis, dystrophy
thyroid function tests thyroid stimulating hormone, TSH	0.5–5 mU/L	low TSH; thyrotoxicosis	tremor, confusion, hyperreflexia
		high TSH; hypothyroidism	apathy, confusion, hyporeflexia, neuropathy

Fig. 13.7 Possible consequences of abnormalities in blood or serum levels of biochemical indices. Individual laboratories may have different normal ranges. (TSH, thyroid stimulating hormone.)

Immunology	
Test	**Associated disorder**
antinuclear factor (ANA)	systemic lupus erythematosus (SLE): fits, confusion, neuropathy, aseptic meningitis, Sjögren's syndrome: gritty eyes, neuropathies, mixed connective tissue disease (MCTD)
anti-double-stranded DNA (dsDNA) antibodies	SLE
rheumatoid factor	rheumatoid arthritis: cervical spine subluxation, neuropathies, vasculitis
anti-Ro (SSA), anti-La (SSB) antibodies	Sjögren's syndrome
antiphospholipid antibodies (e.g. anticardiolipin)	antiphospholipid syndrome
anti-ribonucleoprotein (RNP) antibodies	MCTD; myositis, trigeminal nerve palsies
Jo-1 antibodies	polymyositis
antineutrophil cytoplasmic antibodies (ANCA)	pANCA (peripheral): polyarteritis nodosa cANCA (classical): Wegener's granulomatosis
antiacetylcholine receptor antibodies (AChR)	myasthenia gravis
anti-GM1 antibodies	multifocal motor neuropathy, Guillain–Barré syndrome
anti-GAD antibodies	stiff-man syndrome

Fig. 13.8 Immunology.

Microbiology	
Test	**Associated disorder**
VDRL (venereal disease reference laboratory)	primary syphilis; false positive in pregnancy, systemic lupus erythematosus, malaria
TPHA (*Treponema pallidum* haemagglutination assay)	syphilis; false positive with non-venereal treponemes (yaws, pinta)
hepatitis B surface antigen (HBsAg)	some cases of polyarteritis nodosa
HIV	AIDS

Fig. 13.9 Microbiology.

CSF findings			
Disease	**Protein (g/dL)**	**Glucose**	**Cells**
normal	<0.5	>50% blood glucose	<5/mL lymphocytes, no polymorphs
bacterial meningitis	1.0–5.0	<50%	>1000/mL, polymorphs predominate
viral meningitis	0.5–1.0	normal	<1000/mL, lymphocytes predominate
tuberculous meningitis	1–10	<50%	<1000/mL, lymphocytes predominate

Fig. 13.10 Cerebrospinal fluid findings.

IMAGING OF THE NERVOUS SYSTEM

Plain radiography
Skull radiography
Skull radiography has a limited role in current neurological practice. The main indication is head injury when more sophisticated imaging is not immediately indicated. The standard views are:

- Lateral.
- Postero-anterior.
- Towne's view (fronto-occipital).

Learn the normal skull radiographic markings (Figs 13.11 and 13.12) and the main abnormalities seen on skull radiographs (Fig. 13.13).

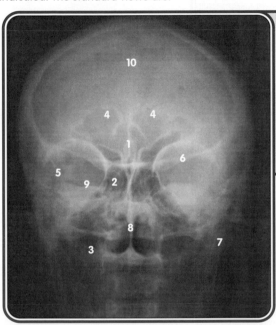

1	crista galli
2	ethmoidal air cells
3	floor of maxillary sinus (antrum)
4	frontal sinus
5	greater wing of sphenoid
6	lesser wing of sphenoid
7	mastoid process
8	nasal septum
9	petrous part of temporal bone
10	sagittal suture

Fig. 13.11 Normal postero-anterior skull radiograph. (Courtesy of J. Weir and P. H. Abrahams.)

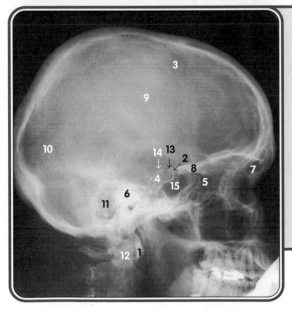

1	anterior arch of atlas (first cervical vertebra)
2	anterior clinoid process
3	coronal suture
4	dorsum sellae
5	ethmoidal air cells
6	external acoustic meatus
7	frontal sinus
8	greater wing of sphenoid
9	grooves for middle meningeal vessels
10	lambdoid suture
11	mastoid air cells
12	odontoid process (dens) of axis (second cervical vertebra)
13	pituitary fossa (sella turcica)
14	posterior clinoid process
15	sphenoidal sinus

Fig. 13.12 Normal lateral skull radiograph. (Courtesy of J. Weir and P. H. Abrahams.)

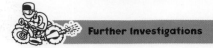

Main abnormalities seen on skull X-ray	
Pathology	**Abnormality**
trauma	skull fractures, intracerebral haematomas (midline shift of a calcified pineal gland)
tumours	bone erosions (metastasis, multiple myeloma) or hyperostosis (meningiomas), calcifications (craniopharyngioma, glial tumours), enlargement/destruction of the pituitary fossa (pituitary tumours)
raised intracranial pressure	separation of the sutures (children), erosion of the posterior clinoids, thinning of the vault, and flattening of the pituitary fossa
developmental defects	craniostenosis, platybasia
inflammatory processes	opacification of the paranasal sinuses
vascular	calcified intracranial aneurysms and vascular malformations

Fig. 13.13 Main abnormalities seen on skull radiograph.

Main abnormalities seen on spinal X-ray	
Pathology	**Abnormality**
trauma	fractures, fracture–dislocations, subluxations
tumours	erosion of the pedicles (long-standing tumours), erosions of the vertebral bodies (metastatic tumours)
degenerative disease	narrowing of disc spaces, calcification of the intervertebral discs, osteophyte formation

Fig. 13.14 Main abnormalities seen on spinal radiograph.

Spinal radiography

The standard views in spinal radiography are:

- Lateral.
- Postero-anterior.

Learn the main abnormalities seen on spinal radiographs (Fig. 13.14).

CT scanning

Using an X-ray source and a series of photon detectors housed in a gantry, computerized tomography (CT) produces a series of consecutive two-dimensional axial brain digital images which show the X-ray density of the brain tissue. The densities of different brain tissues vary according to their X-ray absorption properties, ranging between low (black: air, cerebrospinal fluid) to high (white: bone, fresh blood) (Figs 13.15 and 13.16).

The diagnostic yield of the CT scanning is increased by injecting iodine-containing contrast agents, which enhance the distinction between the different brain tissues and outline the areas of blood–brain barrier breakdown (around tumours or infarctions). Learn the main abnormalities seen on the CT scan (Fig. 13.17)

Magnetic resonance imaging (MRI)

Nuclear magnetic resonance is the term which describes the interaction between the hydrogen protons in the different body structures and strong external magnetic fields. As the patient lies in the scanner, the naturally spinning hydrogen protons align with the strong magnetic field of the scanner. When a further external magnetic field (radiofrequency pulse) of a specific frequency is applied at a right angle, the protons 'flip' out of the main external magnetic field.

As the protons 'relax' back to their original position, they emit a radiofrequency signal that can be digitally analysed and displayed as an image. This 'relaxation' time has two components, known as T1 and T2, which determine the magnetic resonance parameters of the different brain tissues (Figs 13.15 and 13.16).

The paramagnetic agent gadolinium-labelled DTPA (diethylene triamine penta-acetic acid, or pentetic acid) is used as contrast agent. Learn the main abnormalities seen on the MRI (Fig. 13.18).

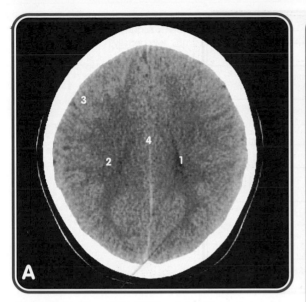

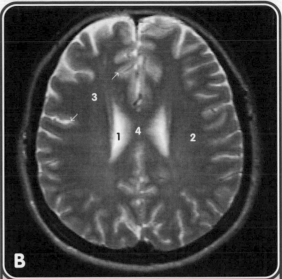

Fig. 13.15 (A) CT and (B) MRI (T2-weighted image) showing the normal structure of the brain.

1	lateral ventricle
2	white matter
3	grey matter
4	corpus callosum

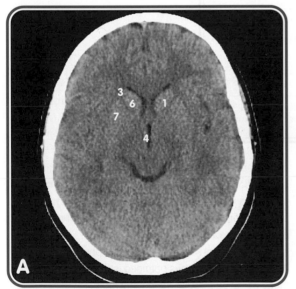

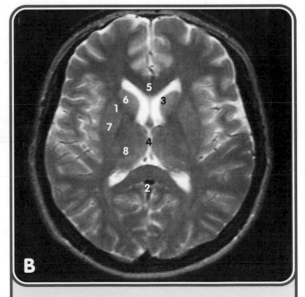

Fig. 13.16 (A) CT and (B) MRI (T2-weighted image) showing the normal structure of the brain.

1	internal capsule
2	vein of Galen
3	frontal horn of lateral ventricle
4	third ventricle
5	genu of corpus callosum
6	head of caudate nucleus
7	putamen
8	thalamus

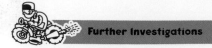

Main abnormalities seen on CT scanning	
Pathology	**Abnormality**
trauma	extracerebral and intracerebral haematomas (HD), brain contusion (mixed HD and LD)
vascular lesions	infarction (LD), haemorrhage (HD), subarachnoid haemorrhage (HD in the basal cisterns and sulci), angiomas, and aneurysms (intensely enhancing lesions)
tumours	enhancing irregular lesions surrounded by LD (oedema)
degeneration	brain atrophy (ventricular enlargement, widening of the sulci, and flattening of the gyri)
hydrocephalus	ventricular enlargement with no evidence of cortical atrophy
infections	abscesses (LD lesions surrounded by ring enhancement), focal encephalitis (LD)
spinal lesions	lesions of the vertebrae, the intervertebral discs, and the spinal canal

Fig. 13.17 Main abnormalities seen on CT scanning. (HD, high density; LD, low density.)

Main abnormalities seen on MRI	
Pathology	**Abnormality**
demyelinating disease	multiple sclerosis (periventricular white matter lesions)
tumours	lesions in the pituitary fossa, cerebellopontine angles, craniocervical junction, and the orbits (images are not affected by artefacts from the surrounding bony structures)
vascular diseases	large aneurysms and venous sinus thrombosis [magnetic resonance angiography (MRA)]
infections	encephalitis, progressive multifocal leucoencephalopathy
spinal lesions	intramedullary lesions (syringomyelia, tumours, demyelination), extramedullary lesions (degenerative disease, tumours, abscesses)

Fig. 13.18 Main abnormalities seen on MRI.

Myelography

A water-soluble iodine-based medium is injected in the subarachnoid space through a lumbar or a cervical approach. This outlines the spinal canal and nerve root sheaths, allowing the assessment of the spinal canal and the nerve roots.

Cord compression caused by extra- or intramedullary lesions is identified as a compression or interruption of the column of contrast.

Postmyelographic CT scanning allows further assessments to the nerve roots within the theca.

Angiography

Serial cranial radiographs are taken after the injection of an iodine-containing contrast agent into a large artery (aorta, carotid, vertebral) to allow the identification of cerebral vessels (Fig. 13.19). Simultaneous digital subtraction of the surrounding soft tissues and bony structures allows the use of more dilute contrast and shorter procedure time, although the spatial resolution of the images will be compromised.

Venous digital subtraction angiography is possible but the quality of the images obtained is distinctly inferior to those obtained through the arterial route.

The indications for angiography are:

- Extracranial atherosclerotic cerebrovascular disease (stenosis, lumen irregularities, or occlusions).
- Aneurysms and arteriovenous malformation.
- Assessing cerebral vessel anatomy and tumour blood supply before neurosurgery.
- Interventional angiography: embolization of angiomas.

Duplex sonography

This technique offers a combination of real time and Doppler flow ultrasound scanning, allowing a non-invasive assessment of extracranial arteries. It is particularly helpful as a screening test for lesions at the carotid bifurcation which avoids the need for angiography in many patients. The quality of this technique is dependent on the experience and skill of the operator.

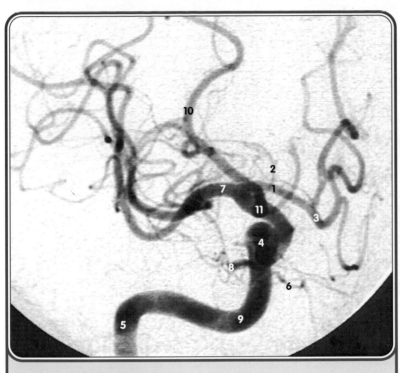

Fig. 13.19 Arterial phase of a normal carotid angiogram. (Courtesy of J. Weir and P. H. Abrahams.)

1	anterior cerebral artery
2	anterior choroidal artery
3	anterior communicating artery
4	cavernous portion of internal carotid artery
5	cervical portion of internal carotid artery
6	ethmoidal branch of ophthalmic artery
7	middle cerebral artery
8	ophthalmic artery
9	petrous portion of internal carotid artery
10	posterior cerebral artery
11	posterior communicating artery

Advantages of MRI
- Absence of ionizing radiation.
- The ability to obtain images in coronal, sagittal, as well as axial plains.
- More sensitive to the pathological changes in the brain tissues.

Disadvantages
- Cannot be used for patients with pacemakers (the magnetic field interferes with their function).
- Cannot be used for patients with ferromagnetic intracranial aneurysmal clips or implants (they distort the images and could be displaced by the strong magnetic field).
- Claustrophobia.

- Describe how you might use plain radiography, CT, MRI, angiography, and myelography to detect a range of diseases.
- What are the basic differences between CT and MRI? What are the advantages of MRI?
- State the contraindications for MRI.

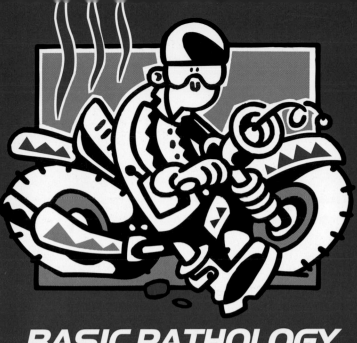

BASIC PATHOLOGY

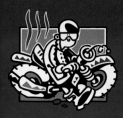

14. The Central Nervous System

Introduction

The bones of the cranium fuse in the first 2 years of life, making the skull a closed structure.

Intracranial pressure is determined by the volume of the three contents of the skull—brain, cerebrospinal fluid (CSF), and blood. None of these three contents is compressible or expandable; therefore, for the intracranial pressure to remain stable, a change in the volume of any of them must be accompanied by an equal and opposite change in the other two. This compensatory mechanism has a limited capacity in terms of speed and magnitude, and its failure results in an increase or decrease in the intracranial pressure (Fig. 14.1).

Cerebral oedema

The skull contains about 900–1200 mL of intracellular and 100–150 mL of extracellular fluid. An increase in the volume of either of these two components results in cerebral oedema.

The pathogenesis of cerebral oedema can be divided into three types—vasogenic oedema, cytotoxic oedema, and interstitial oedema. These types of oedema usually coexist to variable degrees, depending on the primary pathology.

Vasogenic oedema is usually responsive to treatment with corticosteroids, osmotic diuretics, and hyperventilation, whereas cytotoxic oedema is usually resistant to these therapies.

Vasogenic oedema

This is an inflammatory intercellular oedema that results from the increased permeability of the capillary endothelial cells, caused by either defects in the tight endothelial cell junctions or increased active transport, allowing protein-rich plasma to enter the extracellular space.

Such oedema develops around tumours, abscesses and plaques of multiple sclerosis and affects the white matter predominantly.

Cytotoxic oedema

This is an intracellular oedema that results from damage in the ATP-dependent sodium pump, leading to the accumulation of sodium, calcium, and water within the cells (neurons and glia). It affects grey and white matter.

Such oedema is commonly seen in hypoxic brain damage and dilutional hyponatraemia.

Fig. 14.1 Clinical features of raised and low intracranial pressure.

Clinical features of raised and low intracranial pressure		
	Causes	**Symptoms and signs**
raised intracranial pressure	space-occupying masses (e.g. tumour, haematoma, abscess)	early morning headache and vomiting (often without nausea), dizziness, blurred vision, diplopia (usually caused by VI nerve palsy as a false localizing sign), papilloedema, focal sensory and motor neurological signs, depressed consciousness, coma
	increase in brain water content (oedema)	
	increase in cerebral blood flow volume (e.g. vasodilatation, venous outflow obstruction)	
	increased CSF volume (excessive production, impaired absorption)	
low intracranial pressure	decrease in cerebral blood flow volume (e.g. dehydration, blood loss)	headache and nausea mainly on sitting or standing
	decrease in CSF volume (e.g. CSF otorrhoea and rhinorrhoea, lumbar puncture, surgical CSF shunting)	

Interstitial oedema

This is an extracellular oedema seen particularly in hydrocephalus (see later). It results from the extravasation of the cerebrospinal fluid through the ependymal cells into the extracellular space of the periventricular white matter.

Cerebral herniation

The cranial cavity is divided by three rigid barriers—the falx, the tentorium cerebri, and the foramen magnum—into semi-separate compartments (Fig. 14.2). When the intracranial pressure rises because of a space-occupying

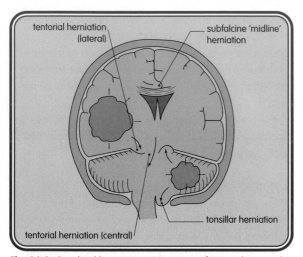

Fig. 14.2 Cerebral herniation. (Courtesy of *Neurology and Neurosurgery Illustrated* by Dr Lindsay *et al.*, Churchill Livingstone, 1991.)

lesion (SOL) in any of these compartments, the surrounding brain tissue is pushed away and forced to herniate into an adjacent cranial compartment, with potentially grave consequences.

Cerebral herniation is divided into four types, as shown in Fig. 14.3.

Hydrocephalus

This is an increase in the cranial cerebrospinal fluid volume. It can be divided into three types:

- Obstructive hydrocephalus: caused by a congenital or acquired obstruction in the cerebrospinal fluid pathway resulting in the accumulation of fluid proximal to the block (Fig. 14.4).
- Communicating hydrocephalus: caused by either increased cerebrospinal fluid production or, more commonly, decreased cerebrospinal fluid absorption (Fig. 14.5).
- Compensatory hydrocephalus: or hydrocephalus *ex vacuo,* which is generalized cerebral atrophy or localized underdevelopment of the cerebrum (porencephaly).

Symptoms and signs of hydrocephalus are given in Fig 14.6. Investigations that may confirm hydrocephalus include the following:

- Skull radiography may show changes suggestive of long-standing hydrocephalus (thinning of the skull vault, enlarged pituitary fossa, and erosions of posterior clinoids).

Types of cerebral herniation		
Clinical type	**Aetiology**	**Clinical signs**
type 1: subfalcine herniation	unilateral hemispheric SOL causing that hemisphere to be compressed beneath the falx	frequently seen radiologically, does not usually cause any clinical signs
type 2: lateral tentorial herniation	unilateral hemispheric SOL causing the uncus of the temporal lobe to herniate through the tentorial hiatus; may progress to type 3	ipsilateral third nerve palsy, ipsilateral hemiplegia (contralateral cerebral peduncle compression)
type 3: central tentorial herniation	midline SOL, very large unilateral hemispheric SOL, or bilateral hemispheric diffuse swelling causing a vertical displacement of the diencephalon through the tentorial hiatus; may progress to type 4	impaired upward gaze (pretectum and superior colliculi compression), hemianopia (occipital lobe infarction), hemi/quadriparesis (cerebral peduncle compression), rising blood pressure and bradycardia (aqueduct compression and hydrocephalus), depressed consciousness and respiration (brainstem compression), coma
type 4: tonsillar herniation	unilateral subtentorial SOL causing herniation of the cerebellar tonsils through the foramen magnum	neck pain, tonic extension of the limbs, cardiac arrhythmia and rising blood pressure, depressed consciousness and respiration, coma

Fig. 14.3 Types of cerebral herniation. (SOL, space-occupying lesion.)

Causes of obstructive hydrocephalus	
Congenital	**Acquired**
aqueduct stenosis	acquired aqueduct stenosis (adhesion following infection or haemorrhage)
Dandy–Walker syndrome	
	intraventricular tumours (colloid cyst, ependymoma)
Arnold–Chiari malformation	
	parenchymal tumours (pineal gland, posterior fossa)
vein of Galen aneurysm	
atresia of fourth ventricle foraminae	space-occupying lesion causing tentorial herniation (see Fig. 14.3)

Fig. 14.4 Causes of obstructive hydrocephalus.

- Head CT scan shows the pattern of ventricular dilatation and excludes the presence of space-occupying lesions.

The treatment of hydrocephalus is as follows:
- Removal of the underlying cause if possible (e.g. tumours).
- Surgical drainage (ventriculoatrial or ventriculoperitoneal shunts).

Causes of communicating hydrocephalus	
Pathogenesis	**Causes**
reduced absorption by arachnoid granulations	infection (especially TB), subarachnoid haemorrhage, trauma, carcinomatous meningitis
excessive CSF production	choroid plexus papilloma
increased CSF viscosity	high protein content

Fig. 14.5 Causes of communicating hydrocephalus.

- **List the features of raised and low intracranial pressure.**
- **Describe the pathogenesis of cerebral oedema.**
- **Name the types of cerebral herniation.**
- **Summarize the pathogenesis and the features of hydrocephalus.**

Fig. 14.6 Symptoms and signs of hydrocephalus.

Symptoms and signs of hydrocephalus		
Age	**Onset**	**Symptoms and signs**
infants and young children	acute	vomiting, depressed consciousness, tense fontanelle, enlarging head, lid retraction and impaired upward gaze, long tract signs
	chronic	mental retardation, failure to thrive, increased skull circumference
adults	acute	signs and symptoms of raised intracranial pressure (see Fig. 14.1), Impaired upward gaze
	chronic: communicating hydrocephalus)	headache and change in mental status
	normal-pressure hydrocephalus	usually in elderly; dementia, gait disturbance, and urninary incontinence

MALFORMATIONS, DEVELOPMENTAL DISEASE, AND PERINATAL INJURY

Neural tube defects

Neural tube defects are caused by varying degrees of failure of fusion of the neural tube and spinal canal. They are geographically variable (e.g. UK>Asia) and multifactorial—environmental and genetic factors appear important. Genetics are complicated in that subsequent children born to a mother with an affected child have a 10-fold increased risk, but monozygotic twins are rarely both affected. Incidence is reduced by taking folate at conception and during early pregnancy.

Spina bifida

The lumbosacral site is most common. Spina bifida is caused by local defects in the development and closure of the neural tube and vertebral arches. The main types are shown in Fig. 14.7.

Deficiency of the meninges in these patients predisposes to meningitis. Bladder problems are also common.

The spinal cord may be tethered by a fibrous band or tight filum terminale, associated with increasing deficit as the child grows and the cord stretches. Surgery to release the tethered cord may therefore be indicated.

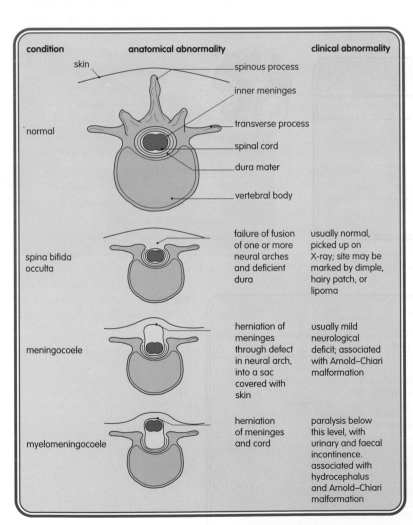

Fig. 14.7 Neural tube defects.

condition	anatomical abnormality	clinical abnormality
normal	skin — spinous process; inner meninges; transverse process; spinal cord; dura mater; vertebral body	
spina bifida occulta	failure of fusion of one or more neural arches and deficient dura	usually normal, picked up on X-ray; site may be marked by dimple, hairy patch, or lipoma
meningocoele	herniation of meninges through defect in neural arch, into a sac covered with skin	usually mild neurological deficit; associated with Arnold–Chiari malformation
myelomeningocoele	herniation of meninges and cord	paralysis below this level, with urinary and faecal incontinence. associated with hydrocephalus and Arnold–Chiari malformation

Anencephaly

Anencephaly represents failure of fusion at the cephalic end of the neural tube. Almost no forebrain structures develop, usually with absence of the skull vault. This condition is not compatible with long-term survival.

Arnold–Chiari malformation

Arnold–Chiari malformation is caused by failure of fusion at the craniocervical junction. The brainstem is displaced downwards, with the cerebellum and cerebellar tonsils descending below the foramen magnum. It is associated with hydrocephalus, especially dilatation of the third and fourth ventricles. It is also associated with lower cranial nerve palsies.

Prenatal diagnosis of neural tube defects

Open spina bifida and anencephaly are detectable prenatally by a raised α-fetoprotein (AFP). The top 3% of maternal serum AFP levels will include most neural tube defects (as well as many normal fetuses, and most twin pregnancies). One in ten pregnant women with a high serum AFP level will have an abnormal baby. Confirmation is with ultrasonography and amniocentesis

Other congenital diseases

Some other congenital diseases are listed below.

- Microcephaly—which can be developmental or caused by intrauterine infection.
- Porencephaly—a focal cyst, which may be asymptomatic and picked up incidentally on CT scan in later life, but often is associated with epilepsy.
- Platybasia—small posterior fossa.
- Arteriovenous malformations—also may be associated with epilepsy or subarachnoid haemorrhage.
- Syringomyelia—a fluid-filled cavity within the cord, sometimes extending to the brainstem (syringobulbia), probably due to many different causes. It is not usually symptomatic until adulthood, when it expands, sometimes provoked by a sudden increase in intracranial pressure (e.g. a fit of coughing). This is rare, but anatomically interesting. The symptoms of syringomyelia are illustrated in Fig. 14.8.
- Diastematomyelia—the spinal cord is split in two, sometimes with a bony spur. Presents as a slowly progressive cord syndrome.

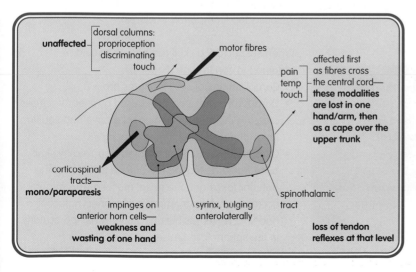

Fig. 14.8 Diagrammatic representation of the cervical cord to explain the symptoms of syringomyelia. Sensory loss is described as dissociated, because pain and temperature sensations are affected, but not joint position and vibration senses. If the cavity extends to the brainstem, dysarthria, dysphagia, tongue wasting, ataxia, and nystagmus may occur.

Cerebral palsy

Cerebral palsy is a heterogeneous group of childhood disorders in which injury to the brain results in a physical neurological disability (Fig. 14.9). Spastic diplegia is most common, sometimes with ataxia, hemiplegia, tetraplegia, and dyskinetic syndrome. Other modalities may also be affected, and there may be associated learning difficulties (although remember that intelligence is frequently preserved), visual problems, and epilepsy. Prevalence is approximately two per 1000 live births.

Prenatal, perinatal, and postnatal causes of cerebral palsy	
Type	**Cause**
prenatal	intrauterine infection (especially TORCH; see p. 197) difficulties in pregnancy; e.g. pre-eclampsia, intracranial haemorrhage
perinatal	asphyxia kernicterus
postnatal	infection respiratory distress syndrome

Fig. 14.9 Prenatal, perinatal, and postnatal causes of cerebral palsy.

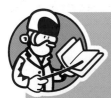

- Describe the types of neural tube defect and the neurological features that may be associated with these.
- Describe the likely presentation of syringomyelia and explain this anatomically.

TRAUMA OF THE CENTRAL NERVOUS SYSTEM

Epidemiology

Approximately 300 per 100 000 of the population require hospital admission annually for head injuries, with an annual death incidence of nine per 100 000. The principal causes include road traffic accidents, falls, assaults, and industrial, domestic, and sports injuries. Alcohol is frequently involved. Although road traffic accidents are the cause of head injury in only 25% of all cases, they contribute to 60% of total fatalities.

Mechanisms

Trauma resulting in brain and spinal cord injuries is of three types:
- Penetrating injuries: e.g. high-velocity missile injuries (gunshot wounds).
- Crush injuries: e.g. industrial injuries.
- Acceleration/deceleration injuries: e.g. road traffic accidents.

Skull fractures

Fractures affecting the vault or the base of the skull are an indication that a significant head injury has occurred. They are of two types:
- Linear fractures.
- Depressed fractures—inner table is depressed by at least the thickness of the skull. The overlying scalp is either intact (simple depressed fractures) or lacerated (compound fractures).

When suspected, a skull radiograph should be obtained to confirm the diagnosis.

Complications of skull fractures are:
- Extradural haematoma—caused by linear fractures crossing the middle meningeal groove and causing the rupture of a meningeal artery.
- Cerebrospinal fluid rhinorrhoea—caused by skull base fractures tearing the dura in the floor of the anterior fossa and the nasal mucosa. This might occasionally be accompanied by pneumatocoeles and fluid levels (visible on radiographs), particularly in the sphenoidal sinuses.

- Cerebrospinal fluid otorrhoea—caused by fractures of the petrous temporal bone.
- Infection—particularly with compound fractures and persistent cerebrospinal fluid fistulae (cerebrospinal fluid rhinorrhoea and otorrhoea), in which case prophylactic antibiotic cover is needed.
- Post-traumatic epilepsy—particularly with compound fractures and dural tears causing cortical scarring.

Parenchymal damage
Primary effect
Loss of consciousness is the hallmark of impact brain damage. This might or might not be associated with structural cerebral damage.

Concussion
This term is often used to describe minor head injuries causing temporary loss of consciousness without macroscopic structural cerebral damage. However, microscopic neuronal damage often occurs. The effect of repeated minor head injury is cumulative: e.g. the 'punch drunk syndrome' in boxers.

Contusion/laceration
The skull and the different parts of the brain have different resistances to the movement induced by the accelerating force. When the head is hit by a moving object (or the moving head hits a static object), the brain is accelerated within the skull, and local brain contusion and laceration (coup) occur, particularly in the undersurface of the frontal and temporal lobes as the brain hits the sphenoidal wing, the petrous temporal bones, and the other non-compliant dural structures. This is usually accompanied by a similar brain injury (contrecoup) at the side directly opposite the local trauma.

Diffuse axonal injury
The combination of linear and rotational acceleration of the brain and the differences in compliance between the white and the grey matter result in tearing of fibres and diffuse axonal injury. This can be identified pathologically by the presence of 'axon retraction balls' and microglial clusters, the number of which depends on the duration of survival and the severity of the head injury.

Secondary effect
Impact brain damage is unavoidable; however, head injury induces other delayed pathological processes, which may be preventable and are potentially treatable. The presenting symptoms of these complications depend on the severity of the initial head injury, but they should be suspected if further deterioration to the level of consciousness occurs or new focal neurological develop.

Intracerebral haemorrhage
Intracerebral haemorrhage arises if arteries or veins crossing the brain tissue are torn. It occurs commonly in the frontal and temporal lobes and is often associated with overlying subdural haemorrhage. In severe head injuries, intracerebral haematoma mixed with necrotic brain tissue might rupture out into the subdural space, giving a 'burst lobe' appearance.

Acute subdural haemorrhage
This is a venous haemorrhage caused by tearing to the superficial veins. It is often associated with damage to the surface of the cerebral hemisphere. Pure subdural haemorrhage with no underlying cortical damage can also occur due to the rupture of the veins bridging from the cortical surface to the venous sinuses.

Extradural haemorrhage
This is an arterial haemorrhage caused by skull fractures tearing the middle meningeal vessels. It usually occurs in the temporal and temporoparietal regions. Such a haemorrhage can occasionally be caused by ruptured venous sinuses.

Subarachnoid haemorrhage
Traumatic subarachnoid haemorrhage occurs in most moderate to severe head injuries. Headache, restlessness, and confusion are the most prominent clinical features. It is often difficult to differentiate between traumatic subarachnoid haemorrhage and aneurysmal subarachnoid haemorrhage complicated by depressed consciousness and subsequent head injury.

Cerebral swelling

Cerebral swelling is a common delayed complication of severe head injuries. It may or may not be associated with intracranial haematoma. The exact mechanism is unknown, but it is often associated with early vasodilatation or an increase in the extracellular or intracellular fluid volume.

Other complications

Other complications are as follows:
- Cerebral ischaemia caused by hypoxia, impaired cerebral perfusion, or delayed vasospasm.
- Tentorial and tonsillar herniation caused by raised intracranial pressure.
- Infection presenting as meningitis or brain abscess in association with compound skull fractures.

Chronic subdural haematoma

Chronic subdural haematoma presents a different clinical picture compared with acute subdural haematoma. It occurs typically in middle-aged and elderly people. A history of high alcohol consumption is common, but a history of head injury is absent in about one-half of the cases. Patients present with headache and fluctuating confusion.

Management

The majority of head injuries are mild and require no specific treatment. In severe head injuries, the principles of management are as follows:
- Adequate airway and oxygenation should be ensured.
- Assessment of associated injuries and treatment of hypovolaemia should be initiated.

Secondary complications should be managed as follows:
- Intracranial haematomas should be treated with appropriate neurosurgical procedures.
- Cerebral swelling should be treated with mannitol, steroids, and ventilation (to maintain low arterial carbon dioxide).
- Antibiotic cover might be indicated.

Neurological sequelae of head injuries

Common neurological sequelae of head injuries are:
- Retrograde and post-traumatic amnesia.
- Focal neurological deficits.
- Post-traumatic epilepsy.
- Postconcussion syndrome.

Post-traumatic epilepsy

The factors associated with a high risk of post-traumatic epilepsy are:
- Seizures in the first week after the head injury.
- Intracranial haematoma.
- Depressed skull fractures, particularly if the dura is torn.

Injuries to the vertebral column and spinal cord

The annual incidence of injuries to the vertebral column and spinal cord is approximately two per 100 000.

In 50% of cases, spinal trauma involves the cervical spine. Injuries to the vertebral column may occur without evidence of cord or spinal nerve injuries; similarly, damage to the neural elements might present without demonstrable injuries to the bone. Neurological damage may result from any of the following four pathological processes:
- Oedema, which occurs early and subsides after a few days.
- Haemorrhage—a degree of haemorrhage into the cord (haematomyelia) is almost a constant feature following major spinal trauma. Haemorrhage into the extradural, subdural, or subarachnoid spaces may also occur and could compress the cord.
- Compression of the cord by fractured or misaligned vertebrae.
- Transection of the cord by elements of the vertebral column.

Clinical features depend on the level of injury and the extent of the lesion. The initial spinal shock (transient suppression of nervous function below the level of injury) begins to subside after a few weeks, and is replaced by spastic weakness.

The principles of management of spinal injuries are:
- Immobilization to prevent further neural damage.
- Preservation of skin integrity (pressure areas).
- Preservation of bladder and bowel function.
- Management of complications (respiratory, cardiovascular, gastrointestinal).
- Long-term rehabilitation.

- ○ **State the incidence of head injury.**
- ○ **What are the complications of skull fractures?**
- ○ **Name the different types of parenchymal brain damage caused by head injury.**
- ○ **What are the mechanisms of neurological damage in spinal injuries?**

CEREBROVASCULAR DISEASE

The risk factors for cerebrovascular disease are as follows:

- Hypertension.
- Diabetes.
- Cardiac diseases: cardiac arrhythmias, rheumatic heart disease, mitral value prolapse, patent foramen ovale, and cardiac myxomas.
- Obesity, hyperlipidaemia, and smoking.
- Alcohol.
- Genetic factors.
- Polycythaemia.
- Other factors: male sex, increasing age, previous cerebrovascular disease, illicit drugs (crack cocaine), antiphospholipid syndrome, and homocystinuria.

Hypoxia, ischaemia, and infarction

There are almost no tissue stores of oxygen or glucose in the brain. When the blood supply fails, the brain ceases to function and cerebral ischaemia/infarction occurs.

The normal cerebral blood flow rate is maintained by a number of haemostatic mechanisms at about 54 mL /100 g/min, which begins to fail when the mean arterial blood pressure falls below a level of 60–70 mmHg.

Progression from reversible ischaemia to infarction depends on the degree and the duration of reduced blood flow. If cerebral blood flow falls below 28 mL/100 g/min this will result in the development of the morphological changes of infarction.

Mechanisms of stroke

There are at least four pathological mechanisms underlying atheromatous cerebrovascular disease:

- Atheromatous changes, particularly in the internal carotid artery immediately above the common carotid bifurcation, act as a source of emboli.
- The atheromatous plaque may reach a size sufficient to stenose or occlude an internal carotid or vertebral artery, compromising the blood flow.
- Occlusion of small (50–150 mm) penetrating branches of the cerebral arteries by plaques of local atheroma or lipohyalinoid degeneration causes small 'lacunar' infarctions distal to the occlusion.
- Lipohyalinoid necrosis and subsequent dilatation of the small intracranial arteries in hypertensive patients causes small miliary aneurysms (Charcot–Bouchard aneurysms) which may rupture, causing intracerebral bleeding.

Lacunar infarctions and Charcot–Bouchard aneurysms occur most frequently in the following sites:

- The putamen and the internal capsule.
- Central white matter.
- Thalamus.
- Cerebellar hemisphere.
- Pons.

It is often very difficult to differentiate clinically between acute cerebral haemorrhage and infarction, and even pathologically between thrombotic and embolic infarctions.

Definitions

- **Transient ischaemic attack** (TIA) is a focal neurological deficit of a presumed vascular origin from which a full clinical recovery occurs within 24 hours.
- **Reversible ischaemic neurological deficit** (RIND) is a focal neurological deficit of a presumed vascular origin from which complete clinical recovery occurs more than 24 hours later.
- **Stroke in evolution** is a focal neurological deficit of a presumed vascular origin which progresses over hours or days.
- **Completed stroke** is a cerebrovascular event with permanent neurological deficit.

Note that persistent asymptomatic neurological signs (e.g. extensor plantars) or imaging abnormalities (CT, MRI) does not exclude the diagnosis of TIA or RIND in otherwise clinically fully recovered patients.

Epidemiology

Cerebrovascular disease is the third most common cause of death after cardiovascular and malignant disease.

The annual incidence of completed stroke in the UK is about 150–200 per 100 000 and the prevalence is about 550 per 100 000.

Clinical features

Transient ischaemic attack (TIA)

TIAs are generally of thromboembolic aetiology. They should be recognized and managed promptly because they are harbingers of strokes. Carotid territory TIAs present with:

- Transient monocular blindness (amaurosis fugax).
- Transient sensory or motor symptoms of the face, arm, or leg.
- Transient aphasia.

Vertebrobasilar TIAs present with a combination of:
- Dysarthria.
- Vertigo and unsteadiness.
- Diplopia.
- Circumoral paraesthesiae.

- Sensory or motor symptoms affecting the limbs singly or in combination.

Stroke

Ischaemic strokes

Thromboembolic infarctions constitute about 85% of all strokes. The clinical features are extremely variable and dependent on the site and the extent of the lesion. Four syndromes can be identified (Fig. 14.10):

- Total anterior circulation infarction (TACI).
- Partial anterior circulation infarction (PACI).
- Lacunar infarction (LACI).
- Posterior circulation infarction (POCI).

Haemorrhagic stroke

Haemorrhagic strokes constitute 15% of all strokes. They are usually caused by rupture of Charcot–Bouchard aneurysms. In the majority of cases, the symptoms develop while the patient is awake and active. Headache is a prominent feature. Clinical features depend on the site of bleeding:

- Capsular haemorrhage: hemiplegia (face, arm, and leg) and depressed consciousness.
- Pontine haemorrhage: tetraplegia, small pupils, and coma.
- Cerebellar haemorrhage: severe headache, ipsilateral ataxia, and depressed consciousness.

Clinical features of ischaemic strokes					
	Clinical features	**Frequency (%)**	**Early mortality**	**Recurrence**	**Functional outcome**
TACI	A combination of: (A) higher cortical dysfunction (aphasia) (B) weakness of at least two-thirds of body areas (face, arm, and leg) (C) homonymous field defect	17	high	moderate	poor
PACI	• two-thirds of the above components • (A) or (B) alone	34	low	high	poor
LACI	• pure motor stroke • pure sensory stroke • sensory motor stroke • ataxic hemiparesis	25	low	moderate	moderate
POCI	• ipsilateral cranial nerve palsy and • contralateral motor or sensory limb deficit • bilateral motor/sensory limb deficit • disorder of conjugate eye movements • isolated cerebellar deficit • isolated homonymous hemianopia	24	low	moderate	moderate

Fig. 14.10 Clinical features of ischaemic strokes.

Investigations

Investigations should be directed towards confirming the diagnosis (CT or MRI scans), or addressing the aetiological factors (electrocardiogram, carotid Doppler, echocardiogram).

Management

In an established stroke, skilled nursing and physiotherapy are the main pillars of treatment. For secondary prevention, all potentially modifiable risk factors should be addressed; aspirin and endarterectomy (for severe symptomatic carotid stenosis) should be considered.

Prognosis

A complete recovery is achieved by 40% of patients; 20% die within 1 month, with 5–10% per year thereafter.

Subarachnoid haemorrhage

Subarachnoid haemorrhage is relatively uncommon. The annual incidence is 10–15 per 1 000 000. Rupture of a cerebral berry aneurysm is the commonest cause (80%), with angiomas accounting for 6% of cases. These aneurysms result from a developmental defect in the media and elastica of the cerebral arteries, causing the media to bulge outward covered only by the adventitia.

Berry aneurysms vary in size (on average, 1 cm) and shape, and are commonly located at the bifurcations of the cerebral arteries (Fig. 14.11). The severity of symptoms is related to the severity of the bleed with:

- Severe headache 'as if I was hit on the head with a sledge-hammer'.
- Nausea and vomiting.

The signs of subarachnoid haemorrhage are:

- Neck stiffness, positive Kernig's sign (pain on passively extending the knee when the hip is flexed to 90°).
- Focal neurological signs (particularly III nerve palsy in posterior communication artery aneurysms).
- Drowsiness, depressed consciousness.

Patients should be investigated with head CT scanning. A lumbar puncture should be performed if the CT scan is normal. Cerebral angiography is essential to locate the aneurysm(s). Patients should be kept in bed and given adequate analgesia. The aneurysm(s) should be clipped neurosurgically at an appropriate time.

Mortality is related to the severity of the bleeding and is particularly high in patients with depressed consciousness.

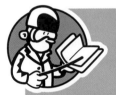

- Discuss the pathological mechanisms of stroke.
- State the differences between TIA, RIND, and stroke, and the different clinical presentations of TIAs and stroke.
- What are the risk factors of cerebrovascular disease?
- What are the causes and the presenting features of subarachnoid haemorrhage?

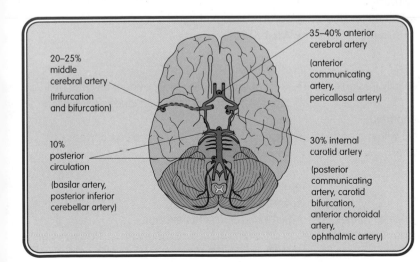

20–25% middle cerebral artery

(trifurcation and bifurcation)

10% posterior circulation

(basilar artery, posterior inferior cerebellar artery)

35–40% anterior cerebral artery

(anterior communicating artery, pericallosal artery)

30% internal carotid artery

(posterior communicating artery, carotid bifurcation, anterior choroidal artery, ophthalmic artery)

Fig. 14.11 Common sites of aneurysms of the intracranial vessels.

INFECTIONS OF THE CENTRAL NERVOUS SYSTEM

Meningitis
Acute bacterial meningitis
Acute bacterial meningitis is an infection of the pia mater and subarachnoid space. The annual incidence in the developed countries is about 5–10 per 100 000. Causative organisms vary with patient age, with three bacteria (NHS) accounting for three-quarters of all cases:

- *Neisseria meningitidis* (meningococcus): 35%.
- *Haemophilus influenzae*: 28%.
- *Streptococcus pneumoniae* (pneumococcus): 16%.
- *Mycobacterium tuberculosis*: 1%.
- Other organisms (staphylococci, other streptococci, *Escherichia coli, Listeria monocytogenes*): 20%.

Clinical features are those of:

- Fever, headache, photophobia, painful eye movements. Impaired consciousness is a late and ominous feature.
- Neck stiffness, positive Kernig's sign.
- Occasionally: petechial skin rash (meningococcal meningitis), focal neurological signs, particularly cranial nerve palsies.

Investigations:

- In the presence of impaired consciousness, or focal neurological signs, head CT scan should be performed first to exclude a space-occupying lesion.
- Lumbar puncture is the key investigation. Cerebrospinal fluid will be turbid with a very high polymorphonuclear count, and low glucose. An immediate Gram stain should be performed and the cerebrospinal fluid should be sent for culture.

Treatment:

- Meningitis is a very serious but potentially treatable condition.
- If the lumbar puncture cannot be performed immediately, prompt 'blind' treatment with a broad-spectrum antibiotic could be life saving.

Prognosis:

- The mortality remains high.
- Overall mortality in the developed countries ranges between 5 and 30%, depending on the causative organism.

Aseptic meningitis
A large number of viruses (mumps, enteroviruses, coxsackie A and B, Epstein–Barr virus) produce an acute self-limiting aseptic meningitis. Patients are moderately ill with fever, malaise, headache, vomiting, and mild neck stiffness. Impaired consciousness is suggestive of an encephalic component (see later).

Cerebrospinal fluid examination shows moderate lymphocytosis. The protein is only slightly elevated, and the glucose is normal. There is no specific treatment, and recovery after few days is the rule.

Intracranial abscess
Intracranial abscesses are rare in developed countries, with an annual incidence of about 0.2–0.3 per 100 000.

Brain abscess
The routes of bacterial invasion are:

- Direct extension from middle ear or sinus infections.
- Haematogenous spread: subacute bacterial endocarditis, right-to-left heart shunts, bronchiectasis.
- Missile penetration of the skull.

Causative organisms are:

- Anaerobic streptococci.
- Bacteroids.
- *Escherichia coli.*
- *Proteus.*
- *Staphylococcus aureus.*

Clinical features:

- Febrile illness.
- Seizures.
- Focal neurological signs.
- Altered consciousness.

Investigations:

- Brain abscesses are readily evident on CT or MRI scans. A characteristic ring enhancement is often seen.
- Evidence of systematic infection (leucocytosis, positive blood cultures).

Treatment:

- Antibiotic therapy.
- Surgical aspiration or excision.

Mortality is high (10–15%).

Extradural (epidural) abscess

Extradural (epidural) abscesses usually result from osteomyelitis of the cranial bone or extension of infection from the frontal or mastoid sinuses. They cause intense local pain and oedema of the scalp.

Subdural abscess

Subdural abscess is a serious complication of paranasal sinus infection or cerebral abscess. It results in cortical vein thrombosis with widespread neurological deficit. Prognosis is grave.

Spinal abscess

Spinal abscess are epidural in two-thirds of cases. One-half of the cases result from haematogenous spread of skin or urinary tract infections, and the remainder from direct spread from vertebral osteomyelitis.
Staphylococcus is the commonest causative organism, followed by *Escherichia coli* and *Proteus*.

Clinical features:
- Severe localized spinal pain.
- Signs of spinal cord compression.

Spinal abscesses should be treated with immediate surgical decompression and antibiotics.

Chronic meningoencephalitis

Tuberculous meningitis

Tuberculous meningitis is uncommon in the developed countries, with an annual incidence of 0.2 per 100 000. It is more common in the socially and economically deprived communities.

Clinical features include:
- Prolonged prodromal illness followed by slowly evolved meningeal symptoms.
- Adhesive arachnoiditis causing cranial nerve palsies and hydrocephalus.
- Localized vasculitis and caseation causing focal neurological signs and seizures.

Investigations:
- Head CT scan should be performed in patients with focal neurological signs or depressed consciousness.
- Cerebrospinal fluid examination shows raised lymphocyte count, high protein, and low glucose.
- Ziehl–Neelsen staining occasionally reveals the presence of acid-fast bacilli, which will be confirmed by culture.

Treatment:
- A combination of isoniazide, rifampicin, and pyrazinamide.
- Pyridoxine is given to prevent isoniazide-induced neuropathy.

Mortality:
- Mortality is very high, reaching 20–30% in treated patients.
- Many survivors are left disabled.

Neurosyphilis

Treponema pallidum (spirochaete) invades the central nervous system within 3–24 months of the primary infection in 25% of untreated cases. Although the incidence of neurosyphilis has declined, it is important to maintain a high diagnostic suspicion since neurosyphilis may mimic other common neurological disorders.

Clinical features include:
- Asymptomatic meningeal neurosyphilis.
- Meningovascular syphilis.
- Tabes dorsalis.
- General paralysis (of the insane).
- Neurosyphilitic gumma (granuloma).

Lyme disease

Lyme disease is a spirochaetal infection caused by *Borrelia burgdorferi*. It presents initially with a characteristic skin rash (erythema chronicum migrans). Fifteen per cent of patients develop neuroborreliosis, which may mimic other common neurological disorders:
- Chronic meningitis.
- Encephalitis.
- Cranial nerve palsies (particularly facial).
- Painful radiculopathy.
- Peripheral neuropathy.
- Mononeuritis multiplex.

Viral encephalitis

Viral encephalitis is an acute febrile encephalitic illness that is often associated with a meningeal component. It can be caused by many viruses, including mumps, herpes simplex and zoster, Epstein–Barr, coxsackievirus, and echoviruses. Herpes simplex encephalitis (HSE) is particularly important because it is treatable.

Clinical features include:
- Headache, fever, altered consciousness.
- Occasionally, acute psychiatric symptoms (delusions, hallucination), seizures, or focal neurological signs.

Investigations:
- Head CT or MRI scans exclude space-occupying lesions and may show focal abnormalities in the affected lobes (particularly the temporal lobe in HSE).
- Cerebrospinal fluid examination shows a raised lymphocyte count, with slightly raised protein and normal glucose, but may be entirely normal.
- EEG shows diffuse slow activity (delta waves), with focal periodic complexes (in HSE).
- Blood and cerebrospinal fluid may show rising viral antibody titres.
- Viruses may be identified in the cerebrospinal fluid (culture, polymerase chain reaction).

Treatment:
- Acyclovir is very effective in HSE. It is relatively non-toxic and should be used whenever this diagnosis is suspected.

Prognosis:
- Varies according to the causative virus.
- If untreated, the overall mortality of herpes simplex encephalitis is about 70%, which can be reduced to 20% with acyclovir.

Other virus-induced neurological diseases

For clinical purposes, viral illnesses are best considered by the clinical syndrome they produce (Fig. 14.12).

Fungal infections

Fungi are frequently the cause of opportunistic infections in immunocompromised patients, particularly in those with HIV. The commonest fungi associated with central nervous system infection in the UK are *Cryptococcus, Nocardia, Candida,* and *Aspergillus.* Fungal infection commonly presents with subacute meningitis complicated by cortical thrombophlebitis and cerebral abscesses. Cerebrospinal fluid examination shows moderate polymorphonuclear leucocytosis, increased protein, and low glucose. The causative fungi can be demonstrated on Gram or Indian-ink staining, or by using special culture techniques.

Treatment is with antifungal agents, but mortality and morbidity are high.

Protozoan infection

Toxoplasma

Toxoplasma gondii is an intracellular protozoan parasite. Humans are occasionally infected through the

Other virus-induced neurological diseases	
Virus	**Neurological syndrome**
varicella zoster virus	shingles

retroviruses
    HTLVI
    HIV
	tropical spastic paraparesis
	AIDS

measles	acute: meningoencephalitis delayed: subacute sclerosing panencephalopathy
rabies virus	rabies
papovaviruses (JC, SV 40)	progressive multifocal leucoencephalopathy
arboviruses	postencephalitic parkinsonism
rubella	congenital rubella
poliovirus	poliomyelitis

Fig. 14.12 Other virus-induced neurological diseases.

ingestion of raw uncooked meat or cat faeces, or by the transplacental route. Congenital toxoplasmosis, caused by transplacental transmission, presents with hydrocephalus, hepatosplenomegaly, retinochoroiditis, and thrombocytopenia.

Acquired toxoplasmosis occurs in immunocompromised patients (particularly in AIDS), with features of meningoencephalitis, seizures, focal neurological signs, and depressed consciousness. Head CT scanning in acquired toxoplasmosis shows characteristic contrast-enhancing lesions.

Toxoplasma immunoglobulin G (IgG) antibodies are found in most patients. Brain biopsy is diagnostic.

Mortality is very high (70%).

Malaria

Cerebral malaria is almost always caused by Plasmodium falciparum. The main clinical features consist of fever and malaise, followed 2–3 weeks later by severe headache, delerium, seizures, progressive stupor leading to coma, and occasionally focal neurological signs.

The diagnosis is established by showing malarial parasites in erythrocytes.

Treatment is with intravenous quinine.

Mortality is high (22%).

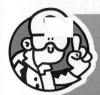

Important prenatal infections associated with neurological sequelae:
T Toxoplasmosis
O Others (Listeria, Salmonella, HIV, syphilis)
R Rubella
C Cytomegalovirus
H Herpes, Hepatitis

Opportunistic infections:
Viruses
 ○ **Cytomegalovirus**
 ○ **Herpes simplex/zoster**
 ○ **JC, SV 40 virus**

Bacteria
 ○ *Listeria*
 ○ *Nocardia*
 ○ *Mycobacterium*

Fungi
 ○ *Cryptococcus*
 ○ *Aspergillus*
 ○ *Candida*

Parasites
 ○ *Toxoplasma*

 ○ **List the clinical features of meningitis and name the commonest causative organisms.**
 ○ **Discuss the clinical features of viral encephalitis.**

DEMYELINATION AND DEGENERATION

Demyelination
Multiple sclerosis
Multiple sclerosis (MS) is a chronic disorder in which episodes of demyelination affect any part of the central nervous system, producing a multiplicity of symptoms. It has an extremely variable course with a tendency towards progressive disability.

Incidence and prevalence
The incidence and the prevalence of MS vary markedly between the different geographical areas and the different population groups. In the UK, the annual incidence is about 5.4 per 100 000, and the prevalence is about 100 per 100 000.

Aetiology
The aetiology of MS is unknown, but is likely to involve environmental factors in genetically susceptible patients. The pathological hallmarks are scattered demyelinating lesions in the perivenous areas of the white matter of the brain and the spinal cord, referred to as 'plaques'.

Symptoms and signs
Depending on the anatomical location of the plaques, four main groups of symptoms are recognized:
- Optic nerve: attacks of optic neuritis presenting with blurring of vision associated with periorbital and retro-orbital pain exacerbated by eye movements, reduced visual acuity, central scotoma, afferent pupillary defect, pink and swollen optic disc (which becomes pale at a later stage).
- Brainstem: diplopia; dysconjugate eye movements, particularly internuclear ophthalmoplegia; limb and gait ataxia, titubation, tremor, dysarthria, and vertigo.
- Spinal cord: sensory symptoms including Lhermitte's phenomenon (electric-shock-like sensation extending down the spine into the limbs on neck flexion); spastic weakness; bladder, bowel, and sexual dysfunction.
- Other clinical features: dementia, euphoria, and emotional lability; facial pain; painful tonic spasms; Uhthoff's phenomenon (transient worsening of symptoms following a hot bath or exercise).

197

Investigation

MS is a clinical diagnosis and no test is pathognomonic. Cerebrospinal fluid shows oligoclonal bands in almost all cases. Evoked potentials (visual, auditory, and somatosensory) could be prolonged. Magnetic resonance imaging is abnormal in almost all patients.

Treatment

Acute relapses are treated with oral or intravenous steroids. Bladder symptoms and spasticity are treated symptomatically. Interferon-β is effective in reducing relapse rate, and might be effective in reducing disease progression.

Prognosis

The average duration of the illness to death is 25–30 years.

Degenerative diseases

Degenerative diseases in which dementia is prominent (cortical dementia)

Alzheimer's disease

Alzheimer's disease is the commonest cause of dementia, accounting for 80% of all cases of dementia in the community. The incidence increases with age; familial cases are occasionally seen. The female:male ratio is 3:1.

Clinical features are those of cortical dementia:
- Memory impairment, apathy, poor reasoning and judgement.
- Aphasia, apraxia, spatial disorientation.
- Eventually patients become mute, bedfast, and incontinent.

The main pathological changes are:
- Considerable brain atrophy, most evident in the superior and middle temporal gyri.
- Neurofibrillary tangles: intracellular paired helical filaments which are particularly common in hippocampal, amygdaloid, and pyramidal neurons.
- Senile plaques: extracellular areas of degenerating neuronal processes surrounding a central core of β-amyloid protein.
- Loss of cholinergic neurons in the medial septal nucleus, the horizontal nucleus, and nucleus of diagonal band.

The cause(s) of Alzheimer's disease is not known, although genetic predisposition is likely to be very important. The high prevalence of Alzheimer's in Down's syndrome suggests that the gene that encodes the β-amyloid precursor, on chromosome 21, is one of the most important candidate genes. Other genes have also been identified.

Investigations, which are largely undertaken to exclude other, treatable, causes of dementia, include:
- Imaging (CT, MRI scans) which, shows brain atrophy, flattening of the gyri, widening of the sulci, and dilatation of the ventricles.
- EEG, which shows non-specific changes; the cerebrospinal fluid is normal.

Treatment:
- There is no effective treatment at present.

Prognosis:
- Most patients die from the complications of immobility within 5–10 years of diagnosis.

Degenerative diseases in which extrapyramidal features are prominent (subcortical dementia)

Parkinson's disease

The annual incidence is 20 per 100 000, with a prevalence of about 190 per 100 000. Age of onset is about 50 years onwards. The cause remains unclear, although genetic and environmental factors [exposure to 1-methyl-4-phenyl-1, 2, 3, 6-tetrahydropyridine (MPTP)] are likely to be important.

The main pathological changes are:
- Loss of the pigmented cells in the substantia nigra which results in severe striatal dopamine deficiency
- Atypical eosinophilic inclusion bodies called 'Lewy' bodies.

Clinical features include the following:
- Bradykinesia is the cardinal feature. Patients present with slowness of gait, difficulties in writing and using their hands, turning in bed, and reduced facial expression.
- Resting tremor classically of four or five cycles per second.
- Rigidity of lead-pipe or (with superimposed tremor) cog-wheeling type.

- Impaired postural control and loss of righting reflexes, causing flexed posture and falls in advanced cases.
- Dementia in 25–50% of cases.

Differential diagnosis:
- Benign essential tremor
- Depression and motor retardation
- Drug-induced parkinsonism
- Other degenerative disorders:
  - Progressive supranuclear palsy (Steel–Richardson–Olzewski syndrome)
  - Multiple system atrophy:
    Shy–Drager syndrome
    Striatonigral degeneration
    Olivopontocerebellar degeneration
  - Diffuse Lewy body disease
  - Alzheimer's disease
- Diffuse cerebrovascular disease with abnormal gait

Investigations:
- The diagnosis is usually based on the clinical features and response to treatment.
- Imaging, autonomic function tests, and sphincter EMG are occasionally needed to exclude other parkinsonian syndromes.

Treatment:
- Anticholinergic and dopaminergic drugs are the main line of treatment.
- Dopaminergic neuronal implantation is still a research procedure.

Prognosis:
- With treatment, life expectancy is now only slightly worse than that of the general population.

Huntington's disease
Huntington's disease is an autosomal dominantly inherited disorder. The gene is on chromosome 4. The prevalence is about 8 per 100 000, and onset is usually in middle age. Pathologically, there is neuronal loss in the striatum associated with deficiency of γ-aminobutyric acid (GABA), acetylcholine, enkephalin, and substance-P.
  Onset is insidious, with:
- Chorea.
- Affective disorder and personality changes.
- Dementia of subcortical type.

Investigations:
- The clinical diagnosis is usually confirmed with genetic studies.
- Head CT and MRI scans in advanced cases show atrophy of the caudate nuclei.

Treatment:
- No specific treatment is available. Chorea is treated symptomatically.
- Genetic counselling of the affected families is essential.

Prognosis:
- Most patients die from aspiration within 10–20 years of diagnosis.

Hereditary ataxias and related disorders
These heterogeneous disorders present with progressive ataxia as a predominant clinical feature (Fig. 14.13).

Motor neuron disease
The annual incidence of motor neuron disease is about 2–3 per 100 000. It usually presents between the ages of 50 and 70 years. Three major types are recognized:
- Amyotrophic lateral sclerosis (ALS): a combination of upper and lower motor neuron limb and bulbar weakness.
- Progressive muscular atrophy: a lower motor neuron limb weakness.
- Progressive bulbar palsy: a combination of upper and lower motor neuron bulbar weakness.

Hereditary ataxias		
hereditary ataxia of known cause	intermittent ataxia	disorder of urea cycle disorders of lactate and pyruvate metabolism (Leigh's disease)
	progressive ataxia	abetalipoproteinuria ataxia telangiectasia xeroderma pigmentosa
hereditary ataxia of unknown cause	spinal ataxia	Friedreich's ataxia
	cerebellar ataxia	pure cerebellar degeneration

Fig. 14.13 Hereditary ataxias.

These syndromes represent a continuum, and patients progress from one syndrome to the other. Sensory symptoms and signs are usually absent. Prognosis is extremely poor and the survival is about 2–3 years.

Spinal muscular atrophy (SMA)

SMA is a group of hereditary conditions characterized by progressive lower motor neuron degeneration. Few distinct phenotypic presentations are recognized:

- Acute infantile SMA (Werdnig–Hoffmann disease).
- Chronic infantile SMA.
- Juvenile onset SMA (Kugelberg–Welander disease).
- Peroneal/scapuloperoneal SMA.

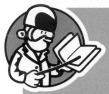

- ○ **What are the clinical features of multiple sclerosis? What is its prevalence?**
- ○ **What are the clinical features of Alzheimer's disease? What is its prevalence?**
- ○ **List the clinical features and the differential diagnosis of Parkinson's disease.**
- ○ **What are the clinical features of Huntington's disease, motor neuron disease, and spinal muscular atrophy.**

METABOLIC DISORDERS AND TOXINS

Vitamin deficiencies

Nutritional vitamin deficiencies are rare in developed countries and are usually seen in chronic alcoholics and socially isolated people, including elderly or mentally ill patients. Vitamin deficiency can also result from diseases (malabsorption, autoimmunity), or drugs (isoniazide), and is usually multiple. Some common features and causes of vitamin deficiences are given in Fig. 14.14.

Vitamin overdose (vitamin A) occasionally results in neurological complications (headache, papilloedema).

Inborn errors of metabolism

Inborn errors of metabolism can be summarized thus:

- Lipid metabolism: e.g. metachromatic leucodystrophy.
- Carbohydrate metabolism: e.g. Pompe's disease.
- Amino-acid metabolism: e.g. phenylketonuria.
- Mucopolysaccharidosis: e.g. Hurler's disease.
- Gangliosidosis: e.g. Tay–Sachs disease.
- Sphingolipidosis: e.g. Niemann–Pick disease.
- Purine and pyrimidine metabolism: e.g. Lesch–Nyhan syndrome.
- Trace metal metabolism: e.g. Wilson's disease.

Mitochondrial cytopathies

These can be classified as either MELAS or MERRF:

- MELAS syndrome (**M**itochondrial **E**ncephalopathy, **L**actic **A**cidosis, and **S**troke-like episodes).
- MERRF syndrome (**M**yoclonic **E**pilepsy, **R**agged **R**ed muscle **F**ibres).

Toxins

Alcohol

Neurological complications of alcoholism include:

- Acute intoxication. The effect of acute alcohol administration depends on the amount of alcohol consumed and on whether the subject is a naïve or chronic alcohol user. The symptoms range in severity from euphoria and mild incoordination to ataxia, dysarthria, and confusion, to deep anaesthesia and respiratory suppression.

- Alcohol withdrawal syndrome (tremors, hallucinations, seizures, and delirium tremens). Action tremor usually reaches a peak 24–36 hours after the cessation of drinking, and is promptly aborted by further alcohol intake. Hallucinations may be visual, auditory, or tactile. Seizures occur 24–48 hours after the cessation of drinking. Delirium tremens combines the three previous features and severe autonomic overactivity (dilated pupils, pyrexia, tachycardia, and sweating).
- Nutritional complications (Wernicke–Korsakoff syndrome and neuropathy). Wernicke–Korsakoff syndrome is caused by thiamine deficiency. Early clinical features are those of ataxia, oculomotor disturbances (oculomotor palsies and nystagmus), and confusion which, if untreated, can progress to coma and death. As the patient's confusion improves following treatment, the amnesic component of the syndrome emerges in which confabulation is a prominent feature. Neuropathy is a symmetrical sensorimotor axonal neuropathy.
- Hepatic complications (acute hepatic encephalopathy and chronic portosystemic encephalopathy).
- Other syndromes: dementia/brain atrophy; alcoholic cerebellar degeneration (characterized by gait and truncal ataxia); alcoholic myopathy (acute painful proximal myopathy); central pontine myelinolysis (acute syndrome of quadriparesis, pseudobulbar palsy occasionally associated with abnormal eye movements and 'locked-in' syndrome).

Carbon monoxide poisoning

The high affinity of haemoglobin to CO results in severe tissue hypoxia. Acute intoxication leads to acute encephalopathy with visual field defects, papilloedema, and retinal haemorrhage. Many patients are left with chronic encephalopathy and parkinsonism.

Clinical features and common causes of vitamin deficiencies			
Vitamin	**Function**	**Cause**	**Neurological sequelae**
A	essential for normal retinal and epithelial cell function	malnutrition	adults and children: blindness infants: mental retardation and hydrocephalus
B$_1$ (thiamine)	pyruvate metabolism	malnutrition, alcoholism	Wernicke's encephalopathy, Korsakoff psychosis, neuropathy
B$_3$ (nicotinic acid)	NAD, NADP coenzyme component	malnutrition	encephalopathy, neuropathy
B$_6$ (pyridioxine)	cofactor in protein metabolism	malnutrition, isoniazide treatment	neuropathy, seizures (infants)
B$_{12}$ (cobalamine)	purine synthesis	autoimmunity, ileal disease, gastrectomy, malnutrition	dementia, myelopathy (subacute combined degeneration), neuropathy
folic acid	purine synthesis	malabsorption, malnutrition	myelopathy, neuropathy, neural tube defect
D	calcium metabolism	malabsorption, malnutrition, chronic renal failure	myopathy
E	antioxidant	malabsorption	cerebellar ataxia

Fig. 14.14 Clinical features and common causes of vitamin deficiencies.

Heavy metals

Lead
Acute encephalopathy is seen largely in children.

Chronic motor neuropathy typically presents with wrist drop.

Mercury
Mercury causes chronic encephalopathy with ataxia, dysarthria, and tremor.

Manganese
Manganese causes chronic encephalopathy and parkinsonism.

Iatrogenic

Drugs
Drug-induced neurological disorders include:
- Encephalopathy: e.g. hypnotics, sedatives, antidepressants in large doses.
- Neuropathy: e.g. isoniazide, vincristine.
- Neuromuscular transmission blockade: e.g. penicillamine.
- Myopathy: e.g. steroids.
- Extrapyramidal syndrome: e.g. antipsychotic medications and antiemetics.
- Psychiatric symptoms: e.g. antiparkinsonian medications.

Neurological complication of opiate abuse:
- ⊙ **Acute intoxication**
- ⊙ **Withdrawal syndrome**
- ⊙ **Transverse myelitis**

- ⊙ **Neuropathy**
  - ⊙ **Acute painful plexopathy**
  - ⊙ **Acute mononeuropathies/ mononeuritis multiplex**

- ⊙ **Myopathy**
  - ⊙ **Rhabdomyolysis**
  - ⊙ **Chronic myopathy**

- ⊙ **Infection**
  - ⊙ **Cerebral abscess**
  - ⊙ **Mycotic aneurysm**

Radiotherapy
Neurological complications are related to the total radiation dose and the period over which it was given. Early features are related to localized oedema. Delayed features are related to necrosis, which often simulates tumour recurrence.

- ⊙ **List the neurological complications of vitamin deficiencies.**
- ⊙ **Describe the neurological complications of alcohol.**

NEOPLASMS OF THE CENTRAL NERVOUS SYSTEM

Primary brain tumours
The annual incidence of primary brain tumours is about 8.2 per 100 000, accounting for about 5% of all neoplasms in the body. The incidence of the different pathological types of primary brain tumours varies from one study to another, but can generally be divided into :
- 56% tumours of glial cells.
- 20% meningiomas.
- 14% pituitary tumours.
- 7% neurinoma.
- 2% medulloblastoma.
- 1% other tumours.

The prevalence of the different tumour types and their anatomical location varies with age:
- Adults: gliomas, metastases, and meningiomas.
    80–85% supratentorial compartment.
    15–20% infratentorial compartment.
- Children: medulloblastomas and cerebellar astrocytomas.
    40% supratentorial compartment.
    60% infratentorial compartment.

The clinical features depend on the site of the tumour and the speed of growth, and can be divided into three main categories:
- Features of raised intracranial pressure (headache, vomiting, and papilloedema).

- Focal symptoms and signs, the nature of which depends on the anatomical site of the tumour and whether the tumour effect is irritative or destructive.
- False localizing signs, e.g. VIth nerve palsy.

Neuroepithelial tumours

Astrocytomas
Astrocytomas are the commonest primary tumours of the brain. They can occur at any age, but are commonest between the ages of 40 and 60. Male/female incidence is 2/1. Astrocytomas occur with equal incidence throughout the frontal, temporal, and parietal lobes, but are uncommon in the occipital lobe.

There are four pathological grades (Kernohan I–IV):
- Low-grade astrocytoma (grades I and II).
- Malignant astrocytoma (grade III).
- Glioblastoma multiformis (grade IV).

Oligodendroglioma
Oligodendroglioma is a slow-growing tumour with low malignancy grade. It affects a younger age-group (30–50 years) and is most common in the frontal lobe. Imaging reveals a well-demarcated tumour, frequently with areas of calcification.

Medulloblastoma
Medulloblastoma is the most common malignant tumour of childhood (4–8 years). It arises from embryonic tissue in the cerebellar vermis and may seed through the cerebrospinal fluid pathways to other parts of the cranium or the spinal cord.

Ependymoma
Ependymoma is the second most common tumour of childhood, although it is also found in the early 20s. It occurs throughout the ventricular system or the spinal canal, but is particularly common in the fourth ventricle and in the caudal part of the spinal cord. Frequently, it infiltrates surrounding tissues. Fourth-ventricle ependymomas usually present with symptoms of intermittent hydrocephalus, ataxia, vertigo, and vomiting.

Meninges

Meningioma
Meningioma is a benign tumour that compresses rather than invades the neural tissues. Maximum incidence occurs between 40 and 60 years of age. It is most common in the sylvian region, the parasagittal surface of the parietal and frontal lobes, the olfactory grooves, the lesser wings of the sphenoid, the tuberculum sellae, the cerebellopontine angle, and the thoracic spinal cord. Imaging reveals a well-circumscribed lesion with occasional calcification.

Nerve sheath cells

Neurofibroma
Neurofibroma is a benign, slow-growing tumour that develops on the vestibular division of cranial nerve VIII. It commonly presents in mid-life and is more common in females. Neurofibroma usually presents with sensorineural deafness, occasionally associated with tinnitus and vertigo.

Anterior pituitary gland

Pituitary adenoma
Pituitary adenoma is a benign tumour that presents with neurological or endocrinological symptoms. Large tumours usually present with headache, bitemporal hemianopia, and occasionally hypopituitarism. Smaller tumours present with hyperprolactinaemia and less commonly with acromegaly/gigantism, Cushing's syndrome, and thyrotoxicosis.

Other tissues
Tumours of other tissues can be summarized thus:
- Blood vessels: haemangioblastoma.
- Germ cells: germinoma, teratoma.
- Microglia: primary brain lymphoma.
- Tumours of maldevelopmental origin: crangiopharyngioma, epidermoid/dermoid cyst, colloid cyst.
- Local extension from adjacent tumours: chordoma, glomus jugulare tumour.

Metastatic brain tumours
The annual incidence of metastatic brain tumour is 8.3 per 100 000. About 20% of patients dying with other tumours will have intracranial metastases, 25% of which are asymptomatic. The primary tumours are:
- 49% bronchus.
- 16% breast.
- 9% bowel.
- 8% genitourinary.
- 18% others.

Presenting features are similar to those of the primary brain tumours.

Investigations of brain tumours

Investigations are aimed to identify the presence of the tumour, its anatomical site, and its pathology with:

- Imaging (CT, MRI, angiography).
- Biopsy.

Treatment

Treatment depends on many factors, mainly the type, site, and stage of the tumour, and includes:

- Symptomatic: analgesia, steroids.
- Specific: surgery, radiotherapy, chemotherapy.

Prognosis

The great majority of patients with cerebral tumours have a limited life expectancy, with a median survival of a few months. More benign tumours allow survival for many years.

- **State the prevalence of the different types of primary brain tumours according to age and anatomical location.**
- **List the main types of benign and malignant primary brain tumours.**
- **State the incidence of metastatic brain tumours.**

Effects of systemic cancer on the central nervous system:
- **Direct invasion from adjacent structures**
- **Metastatic disease**
- **Non-metastatic 'remote effect' (paraneoplastic syndromes)**
    - **Immunologically mediated: Cerebellar dysfunction Visual dysfunction Sensory neuropathy Opsoclonus**
    - **Lambert–Eaton myasthenic syndrome**
    - **Limbic encephalitis**
- **Others (opportunistic infections, dermatomyositis, inappropriate ADH secretion)**

EPILEPSY

An epileptic seizure (fit) is a paroxysmal alteration in nervous system activity that is time limited and causes a clinically detectable event. The types of epileptic seizure are given in Fig. 14.15.

Epilepsy is a condition in which more than one seizure has occurred. Incidence is greatest in early and late life, with a prevalence of about 6 per 1000.

Febrile convulsions in childhood are not classed as epilepsy, although, if prolonged, these may predispose to epilepsy in later life.

Epilepsy is a clinical diagnosis and the patient is often normal on examination; therefore a careful history is vital. It is particularly useful to obtain a history from a witness to the seizure.

A patient who has had a seizure with loss of consciousness may remember feeling odd (e.g. odd smells, metallic taste) before the event (the aura), and may remember feeling confused and disorientated afterwards (the postictal phase), but will have no memory of the fit itself. Surprisingly, perhaps, tongue-biting, and urinary incontinence are infrequently seen.

Risk of another seizure within 1 year of the first is 40%, rising to 50% within 3 years.

Status epilepticus is defined as two or more seizures in succession without recovery between, or a seizure lasting longer than 30 minutes. This is a medical emergency, requiring immediate hospital admission and treatment.

Partial (focal) epilepsy

Focal epilepsy may arise from an intracerebral structural defect, causing motor or sensory symptoms localized to one body part, which may then spread to adjacent areas as the electrical activity spreads to contiguous regions of the cortex (e.g. jacksonian seizure): simple partial seizures. Sometimes, no underlying structural defect can be found.

Complex partial seizures usually arise in the temporal lobe. They are called 'complex' because they are associated with disturbance of consciousness.

Seizures arising in the medial temporal lobe may produce disturbances of smell and taste, visual hallucinations, and a sense of *déjà vu*. These may evolve to a tonic–clonic seizure (secondary generalization). Weakness following the event may occur for minutes or hours (Todd's paresis).

Primary generalized epilepsy

Any of the seizure types indicated in Fig. 14.15 may occur in one patient. In a generalized tonic–clonic seizure, the tonic ('increased tone') phase is a sudden tonic contraction of muscles usually with upward eye deviation. The clonic ('with clonus-type activity') phase follows. Initial EEG changes are often bilateral. This condition usually has its onset in childhood. Absence (or petit mal) attacks usually consist of a brief interruption of activity, sometimes with complex motor activity (such as fumbling with clothes), but without collapse. EEG during this event shows a three-per-second spike-and-wave activity (Chapter 13, Fig. 13.2).

Epilepsy syndromes

The International League Against Epilepsy classifies certain conditions as epilepsy syndromes, which includes clinical and EEG manifestations. These include:

- Benign childhood epilepsy with centrotemporal spikes.
- Lennox–Gastaut syndrome.
- Infantile spasms.
- Juvenile myoclonic epilepsy (JME): a familial late childhood onset disease, with myoclonic jerks, tonic–clonic seizures ± absence seizures, with typical interictal EEG.

Pseudoseizures

Pseudoseizures (simulated seizures) occur in up to 20% of patients referred for 'intractable epilepsy'. They may occur in association with real epilepsy.

Investigation

This includes EEG (Chapter 13) (remember, about 50% are normal and this does not disprove the diagnosis), CT, and/or MRI in adult-onset seizures, with further investigation as appropriate to the individual.

Fig. 14.15 Types of epileptic seizure.

Types of epileptic seizure	
primary generalized epilepsy	absence seizures; primary generalized tonic–clonic seizures; others: myoclonic, atypical absences; tonic, clonic and atonic seizures
partial (focal) epilepsy ± secondary generalization	simple partial seizure (without loss of consciousness), complex partial seizures (with disturbed consciousness)
secondary generalized epilepsy	due to underlying generalized cerebral abnormality
epilepsy due to underlying focal or metabolic cause	primary intracranial lesions (tumour, stroke, infections, trauma), metabolic (hypoglycaemia, hypomagnesaemia, liver failure), drugs (and most in overdose), drug withdrawal (alcohol, benzodiazepines), toxins (alcohol, carbon monoxide)

Treatment

First fits are often not treated, but unless seizures are years apart, most neurologists would treat after the second event. There are a wide range of antiepileptic medications, and choice depends mostly on seizure type. A major reason for differentiating partial from generalized seizures is that different drugs are effective for each. Some patients with suitable seizure activity may benefit considerably from surgical removal of an epileptogenic focus on a temporal lobe.

Epilepsy and driving
First fit/solitary fit
○ 1 year off driving (fit free) with medical review before restarting. If another fit occurs during this time, the patient must wait a year from that fit before review.

Loss of consciousness without known cause
○ As above.

Seizures during sleep
○ After one seizure, regulations as above. If all attacks for at least 3 years have been during sleep, and the patient has never had an awake attack, driving is allowed.

Withdrawal of antiepileptic medication
○ Advise not to drive (but not a legal obligation on the patient's part) for 6 months from time of withdrawal. Clearly, if further seizures occur, the above regulations apply.

Factors that may stimulate seizures:
○ Sleep
○ Sleep deprivation
○ Drugs (which may 'lower the fit threshold')
○ Intercurrent illnesses
○ Reflex causes (e.g. flashing lights, computer screens, startle, loud noise)
○ Stress

○ Describe how you would identify that a patient has had an epileptic seizure.
○ How is epilepsy defined?
○ What would you advise a patient who has had three fits in a month, with regard to driving?

DISEASES OF THE AUTONOMIC NERVOUS SYSTEM

Causes of autonomic failure
These may be generalized or focal.

Generalized
There are three groups of generalized autonomic disease: central, peripheral, and drugs.

Central
Central causes of autonomic failure are:
- Multiple system atrophy (especially Shy–Drager syndrome).
- Parkinson's disease.
- Progressive autonomic failure.
- Central brain lesions (tumour, vascular, infection).
- Acute spinal cord disease.

Peripheral
Peripheral neuropathies that may have pronounced autonomic features include:
- Diabetes.
- Amyloid neuropathy.
- Guillain–Barré syndrome.
- Alcoholic neuropathy.
- AIDS.
- Vincristine neuropathy.
- Hereditary sensory and autonomic neuropathy, Fabry's disease, Tangier disease.
- Botulism.

Drugs
The following drugs in particular may have autonomic side effects:
- Antidepressants.
- Vasodilators.
- ACE (angiotensin-converting enzyme) inhibitors.

Focal
Focal autonomic symptoms may be due to:
- Horner's syndrome (Figs 14.16 and 14.17).
- Parasympathetic disturbance of the eye: cranial nerve III palsy or tonic (Holmes–Aidie) pupil; the latter is a dilated pupil in association with reduced tendon reflexes.
- Phaeochromocytoma.
- Lumbar sympathectomy.

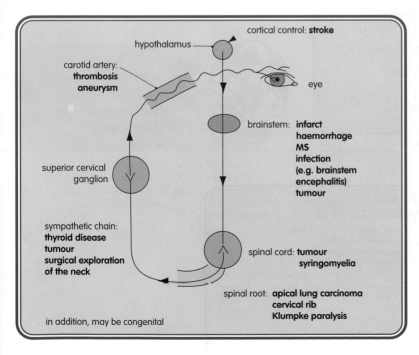

Fig. 14.16 Causes of Horner's syndrome. Arrows indicate a representation of the course of the sympathetic pathways. Bold type indicates possible pathologies at each level.

- Infiltrating lesions of the parasympathetic, sacral plexus.
- Acute spinal cord lesions.

Multiple systems (or multisystem) atrophy

Multiple system atrophy is a term coined in the late 1960s to describe a group of three overlapping conditions with associated neurodegeneration, as outlined in Fig. 14.18. Therefore, most patients will eventually have features of all three. Pathologically, characteristic argyrophilic cytoplasmic inclusion bodies are seen in oligodendrocytes and neurons that appear to be tangles of microtubules. Pathological, positron emission tomography (PET) and clinical studies have confirmed the unity of these syndromes, which seem to be varying phenotypes of the same underlying disease process.

Parkinsonism in these disorders is only slightly, or not at all, responsive to treatment. Symptoms begin in middle age and usually progress to death in a few years.

Prominent autonomic features of Shy–Drager syndrome include:

- Postural hypotension.
- Impotence.
- Urinary problems (retention or incontinence).
- Constipation.
- Decreased sweating, dry eyes, and dry mouth.
- Decreased pupillary responses to light.

There is no treatment for the underlying neurodegeneration, but autonomic symptoms may be helped by simple measures such as a head-up tilt at night, and by drugs such as intranasal desmopressin or fludrocortisone.

Progressive autonomic failure

Progressive autonomic failure occurs in middle age, and men are affected twice as often as women. Impotence and loss of libido are commonly presenting symptoms in men. Postural dizziness and bladder symptoms usually follow.

Horner's syndrome: effects	
Lesion beyond superior cervical ganglion (peripheral)	**Lesion before superior cervical ganglion (central)**
partial ptosis miosis enophthalmos	partial ptosis miosis enophthalmos
may not affect sweating	anhidrosis
pupil constricts with adrenaline drops	no effect (as normal pupil)

Fig. 14.17 Effects of Horner's syndrome.

- **What is Horner's syndrome and what are its causes?**
- **What is multiple systems atrophy?**

Fig. 14.18 Conditions comprising multiple systems atrophy.

Conditions comprising multiple systems atrophy			
Syndrome	**Prominent sign**	**Additional signs (usually presenting later)**	**Pathology**
Shy–Drager syndrome	autonomic failure	parkinsonism	cerebellar, nigral, and striatal pathology
striatonigral degeneration	parkinsonism	autonomic and cerebellar	degeneration of corpus striatum and substantia nigra
olivoponto-cerebellar atrophy (OPCA)	ataxia	autonomic and parkinsonism	atrophy of olive, pons, and cerebellum

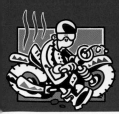

HEREDITARY NEUROPATHIES

Hereditary motor and sensory neuropathies (HMSNs)

These include all inherited neuropathies that affect both the motor and sensory peripheral nerves. Incidence is about 1/2500. Classification is changing as molecular genetic defects are discovered. No treatments are yet available, but much can be done in terms of helping the patient overcome his or her disability. Distal wasting and weakness ('inverted champagne-bottle legs'), areflexia, pes cavus and claw toes, and distal sensory loss are characteristic.

HMSN I

This is also still called Type 1, or hypertrophic (describing the histological appearance of the nerves) Charcot–Marie–Tooth (CMT) syndrome. It is usually autosomal dominant:

- Type a: usually caused by a duplication on chromosome 17 (c17), which includes the gene for *PMP22*, a peripheral nerve myelin protein.
- Type b: caused by mutations on c1, including the gene for *P0*, another myelin protein.

Autosomal recessive and X-linked inheritance also occur, the latter associated with mutations in the gene for *connexin 32*, a gap-junction protein.

Because myelin genes appear to be affected, it makes sense that this is a 'demyelinating neuropathy', and nerve conduction velocities are slow. The age of onset is usually the first or second decade, but sometimes it is much later.

Symptoms vary greatly: up to 20% of those affected are significantly disabled as adults, but a similar proportion are asymptomatic.

HMSN II

This is also still called Type 2, or neuronal CMT syndrome. This is an 'axonal' neuropathy (i.e. with relatively preserved nerve conduction velocity, but small motor and sensory action potentials). It is usually autosomal dominant, in some cases linked to c1.

HMSN III

This is also called Déjérine–Sottas disease. It is more severe, presenting in infancy. Recent molecular discoveries indicate that these cases may be 'severe HMSN I'.

HMSN IV

This is also called Refsum's disease (a more useful name probably as this is a distinct clinical entity). Metabolic defects occur in phytanic acid metabolism, hence this acid accumulates. Features include sensorineural deafness, ataxia (caused by cerebellar degeneration), retinitis pigmentosa, anosmia, ichthyosis (scaly, thickened skin), cataracts, cardiomyopathy, and skeletal deformities (short forth and fifth fingers and toes).

The condition may respond to a diet low in phytanic acid.

Other HMSNs

- HMSN V: with pyramidal signs.
- HMSN VI: with optic atrophy.
- HMSN VII: with deafness.
- HMSN VIII: with pigmentary retinopathy.

Hereditary sensory neuropathy

This is a rare autosomal recessive or dominant condition that usually presents in childhood. Loss of pain occurs (predominantly) in the hands and feet. Charcot joint deformities and neuropathic ulcers of the feet also appear.

- **HMSN I is a demyelinating neuropathy with slow conduction velocities.**
- **HMSN II is an axonal neuropathy with near-normal conduction velocities.**
- **HMSN III presents like an early-onset, severe HMSN I.**

There is no treatment as such; however, the patient may be helped by the doctor in many ways.

Hereditary sensory and autonomic neuropathy

This is also called Riley–Day syndrome and is rare. Aplasia of peripheral autonomic neurons occurs. Symptoms include absence of tears, abnormal sweating, fevers, skin blotching, sensory neuropathy, and poor blood-pressure control.

Treatment that aims to aid symptoms (e.g. fludrocortisone to aid postural hypotension) may be useful.

Other inherited neuropathies

Hereditary neuropathy with liability to pressure palsies (HNPP) is an autosomal dominant condition caused by a deletion of the same region of c17 that is duplicated in HMSN Ia.

All the other inherited neuropathies are very rare, for example:

- Fabry's disease.
- Metachromatic leucodystrophy.
- Tangier disease.
- Porphyria.

- A patient presents with weak, wasted lower legs. His sister and father are similarly affected. Discuss possible causes.

TRAUMATIC NEUROPATHIES

Trauma to a nerve causes weakness or numbness in the area supplied by that nerve, although sensory nerve injuries tend to cause symptoms and signs in an area smaller than that which the nerve supplies, owing to overlap in sensory territories. Trauma may partially or completely disrupt the nerve's function. Types of nerve injury are given in Fig. 15.1. Axons regrow at a rate of 1.0–1.5 mm/day.

Compression neuropathy
Carpal tunnel syndrome

Carpal tunnel syndrome is common, especially in women. It is caused by pressure on the median nerve as it passes deep to the flexor retinaculum at the wrist. Initial symptoms are pain and tingling in the median nerve territory (most commonly the index and middle fingers), characteristically at night, causing the patient to shake the hand over the side of the bed for relief. Sometimes the pain shoots up the arm from the wrist. Signs are often missing at this stage but, as often in neurology, the history is the clue. With time, median nerve innervated muscles, especially abductor pollicis brevis, may become weak and wasted and sensory signs may be found (Fig. 15.2).

Tinel's sign (tapping over the wrist) and Phalen's test (flexing the wrist for a minute) may reproduce symptoms, although they are not particularly useful in practice, especially if a careful history has been taken. Predisposing factors for carpal tunnel syndrome are given in Fig. 15.3. The diagnosis may be confirmed with nerve conduction studies.

Treatment may be non-surgical (wrist splints in slight extension, or local steroid injection) or surgical (decompression).

'Saturday night' palsy

'Saturday night' palsy is caused by compression of the radial nerve, especially if an arm is draped over a chair for some hours. Wrist drop and weakness of finger extension occur, but not usually sensory loss (because of sensory overlap and because the posterior cutaneous nerves arise above the elbow). Patients usually recover spontaneously in a few months.

Ulnar nerve compression

This usually occurs at the elbow (in the groove of the medial epicondyle), particularly during general anaesthesia, with the use of crutches, and secondary to previous elbow injury. It can also occur in the cubital tunnel (the fibrous band between the heads of flexor carpi ulnaris). Symptoms include pain along the medial aspect of the forearm and numbness in the little and ring fingers, with wasting and weakness of ulnar-innervated small hand muscles, especially the first dorsal interosseous muscle. If the branch to flexor digitorum profundus is affected (in lesions above the cubital tunnel) there will also be weakness of flexion of the distal interphalangeal joint.

Treatment involves avoiding unnecessary trauma to the nerve (no leaning on the elbows) and sometimes surgery.

Meralgia paraesthetica

This is a syndrome of tingling, pain, and numbness on the anterolateral surface of the thigh caused by compression of the lateral cutaneous nerve of the thigh under the lateral end of the inguinal ligament. It is more common in the obese, in pregnancy, and with very tight trousers.

Treatment, other than weight reduction and sartorial reconsideration, is unnecessary.

Cervical spondylosis

Cervical spondylosis may cause compressive injuries of cervical roots as they pass through their foramina. The roots of C5, C6, and C7 are commonly affected.

If C5 and C6 roots are affected, there may be depression or absence of the biceps and supinator reflexes, with exaggeration of the triceps reflex.

Avulsions

Avulsion of the spinal roots is generally caused by severe traumatic injury. The two basic types are:

- Erb paralysis: caused by avulsion of C5 and C6 roots because of pressure on the shoulder, usually after motor cycle accidents or, in babies, after forceps delivery. The shoulder cannot be abducted and the elbow cannot be flexed, therefore the arm hangs limply.
- Klumpke paralysis: avulsion of C8 and T1, usually occurring when the arm is pulled forcibly upwards. Loss of function affects the small muscles of the hand and the long finger flexors and extensors, so the hand has no useful function.

Lacerations

Penetrating injury and fracture may lacerate a nerve, causing loss of function in the territory it supplies.

- Ulnar nerve: usually at the elbow, causing signs as above.

Fig. 15.1 Types of nerve injury.

Types of nerve injury		
Neuropraxia	**Axonotmesis**	**Neurotmesis**
transient block	damage to axon, preserved nerve sheath	complete section of a nerve
no microscopic evidence of nerve degeneration; nerve function is partially disrupted; recovery is rapid	Wallerian degeneration; nerves regrow in sheath; effects on function may be severe, but recovery occurs	Wallerian degeneration; paralysis/sensory loss are complete; vascular and trophic changes occur

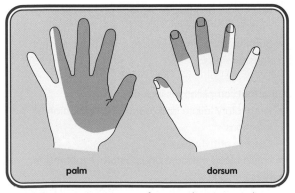

palm   **dorsum**

Fig. 15.2 Approximate area of sensory loss in a median nerve lesion.

Predisposing factors for carpal tunnel syndrome
arthritis of the wrist obesity pregnancy hypothyroidism and acromegaly hereditary neuropathy with liability to pressure palsies (HNPP) repetitive wrist movements (washing floors, vibrating tools)
But it is usually idiopathic!

Fig. 15.3 Predisposing factors for carpal tunnel syndrome.

- Median nerve: with fractures in the arm, resulting in weakness of forearm flexors, flexor digitorum profundus (the patient cannot flex the distal interphalangeal joint of his forefinger), and commonly abductor pollicis brevis, together with sensory loss as shown in Fig. 15.2. Note that a compression (between the two heads of pronator teres) or traumatic injury affecting the anterior interosseous nerve causes loss of flexion of the distal interphalangeal joints of the thumb, index finger, and sometimes middle finger, without sensory loss.
- Radial nerve: with fractures of the shaft of humerus, causing a similar picture to Saturday night palsy.
- Femoral nerve: femoral artery cannulation may rarely result in damage.
- Sciatic nerve: may be damaged with fractures of the femur and pelvis, misplaced intramuscular injections or penetrating injury.

Vertebral and spinal cord segmental levels:
There are seven cervical vertebrae and eight cervical cord segments.
The spinal cord ends at the vertebral body of L2, therefore the spinal segments must 'fit in' above this.

Vertebral body	Spinal cord segment
C7	C8
T10	T12
T11	L1–2
T12	L3–4
L1	L5
L2	S1–5

° **Describe the features of carpal tunnel syndrome.**
° **How may a nerve be damaged and what would you expect clinically?**

Guillain–Barré syndrome (GBS)

This is a clinical syndrome caused by an acute peripheral neuropathy, affecting motor more than sensory nerves, and in most cases following infection. The incidence is about 2/100 000. Following the illness, 20% of patients remain so disabled that they are unable to work after a year, and 5% die. By definition, the illness progresses for less than 4 weeks. About half the patients recall a preceding diarrhoeal illness or upper respiratory tract infection a few days or weeks before neurological signs develop. Preceding infections include:

- *Campylobacter jejuni.*
- Influenza.
- Epstein–Barr virus and cytomegalovirus.
- Herpes zoster virus.
- Hepatitis.

Preceding immunization has also been implicated.

In most cases, there is inflammation and demyelination—acute inflammatory demyelinating polyradiculopathy (AIDP)—and the nerves may recover by remyelination. In about 5%, the same clinical picture (i.e. syndrome) may be produced by an acute motor or acute motor and sensory axonal neuropathy (AMAN and AMSAN), where the brunt of the injury falls on the axons primarily, and the potential for spontaneous recovery may be less.

The clinical features are:

- Development of symptoms over days or weeks.
- Bilateral flaccid weakness (and later wasting) of proximal and distal limb muscles.
- Loss of tendon reflexes.
- Progression of weakness in some cases to affect the respiratory and bulbar (speech and swallowing) muscles.
- Burning pains and numbness, but often without sensory signs.

Important complications include:

- Respiratory failure and associated respiratory infections.
- Cardiac arrhythmias.
- Labile blood pressure and postural hypotension.
- Pressure sores.
- Anxiety and depression.

Investigations:
- In AIDP in particular, nerve conduction studies show slowing of conduction velocities. Action potentials are often reduced.
- Cerebrospinal fluid protein is usually raised (up to 5 g/dL), but the cell count is normal.

The Miller–Fisher syndrome is a variant of GBS with:
- An eye movement disorder caused by cranial nerve III, IV, or VI palsies.
- Cerebellar ataxia.
- Areflexia.

Management involves avoidance of complications, by regular measurement of the vital capacity (deterioration may be rapid; the patient may require ventilation only hours after symptoms begin), constant electrocardiogram recording, and careful nursing. Plasma exchange and intravenous immunoglobulin are equally effective at hastening recovery.

Differential diagnosis of Guillain–Barré syndrome

Neuropathies:
- Porphyria.
- Acute heavy metal poisoning.
- Diphtheria.
- Vasculitis.
- HIV-related neuropathy.

Anterior horn cell:
- Poliomyelitis.

Central nervous system:
- Cord compression.
- Transverse myelopathy.
- Brainstem infarction.

Neuromuscular:
- Myasthenia gravis.
- Botulism.

Muscular:
- Periodic paralysis.
- Acute polymyositis.

Chronic inflammatory demyelinating polyradiculopathy (CIDP)

CIDP has a similar pathology to AIDP, but it follows a relapsing–remitting course, with more slowly progressive onset of signs.

The condition responds to steroids, intravenous immunoglobulin, and plasma exchange.

Paraproteinaemic neuropathy

Paraproteinaemic neuropathy is associated with:
- Monoclonal gammopathy of undetermined significance (especially with IgM and IgG paraproteins).
- Multiple myeloma (especially osteosclerotic).
- Solitary plasmacytoma.
- Waldenström's macroglobulinaemia.

Other inflammatory neuropathies

These include:
- Vasculitides: non–systemic vasculitic neuropathy, systemic vasculitis of any cause (e.g. polyarteritis nodosa, systemic lupus erythematosus, lymphoma).
- Sarcoidosis.
- Diphtheritic neuropathy (the exotoxin causes demyelination by interfering with cell function; the bacteria do not invade the nerve).
- Lyme disease (Bannwarth's syndrome).
- AIDS.

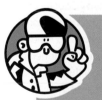

Causes of multiple mononeuropathy:
- **Collagen vascular disease (e.g. systemic lupus erythematosus, rheumatoid arthritis, Sjögren's syndrome, polyarteritis nodosa).**
- **Diabetes mellitus.**
- **Sarcoidosis.**
- **Infections (e.g. Lyme disease, leprosy, AIDS).**
- **Paraneoplastic syndromes.**
- **Alcohol.**
- **Hereditary neuropathy with liability to pressure palsy.**

INFECTIOUS NEUROPATHIES

Postinfectious neuropathies

These include:

- Guillain–Barré syndrome (p. 212).
- Diphtheria: rare in the UK. Progressive peripheral neuropathy caused by the exotoxin, may occur a few weeks after the acute febrile illness. Supportive treatment until recovery is necessary.
- Lyme disease (Bannwarth's syndrome): rare in the UK. Caused by infection by *Borrelia burgdorferi,* a spirochaete, transmitted by *Ixodes* ticks. A Guillain–Barré-type syndrome may occur some weeks later. Treatment of the acute illness is with benzylpenicillin; the subsequent neuropathy recovers gradually.

Infectious neuropathies

These are all rare in the UK. They include:

- Leprosy: common in endemic regions. Causes a patchy peripheral neuropathy (motor and sensory loss) with hypopigmented, anaesthetic skin lesions and thickened nerves. Diagnosis is by skin or nerve biopsy; the acid-fast bacilli are seen within the tissue.
- Tetanus: caused by infection of a wound by *Clostridium tetani.* Days to weeks later, rigidity and pain in voluntary muscles occur, with difficulty opening the jaw (trismus), facial stiffness (risus sardonicus), dysphagia, back stiffness hyperextension, and respiratory difficulty. Treatment includes debriding, benzylpenicillin, human antitetanus immunoglobulin and good supportive care in a quiet environment (because stimulation may induce spasms).
- Botulism: caused by ingestion of *Clostridium botulinum.* A neurotoxin may cause a symptoms because of cholinergic blockade. Hours to days later, lower motor neuron and autonomic symptoms may occur, with flaccid weakness spreading to include respiratory muscles. This may mimic myasthenia

gravis or Guillain–Barré syndrome. Antitoxin and penicillin treat the acute infection but are probably not effective once neurological signs are present, so good supportive care is necessary whilst awaiting recovery.

- Herpes simplex (type 2) virus: may cause lumbosacral radiculitis.
- Herpes zoster virus: 'shingles', or a recrudescence of latent herpes zoster which has remained dormant in the dorsal root ganglia since an attack of chickenpox in earlier life, may occur in normal people, but is more common in the immunosuppressed (especially those with haematological malignancies and AIDS). The typical rash is usually present. Symptoms caused by peripheral nerve involvement include pain, then numbness in the area of the rash, flaccid weakness in the root distribution of the rash, which may then spread, and Guillain–Barré syndrome. Other neurological sequelae of herpes virus infections include encephalitis, transverse myelitis, and a middle cerebral artery vasculitis. Intravenous acyclovir is the treatment for all neurologically serious complications of herpes virus infections.
- HIV: may present with a variety of neurological manifestations. Acute complications include mild viral meningitis at the time of seroconversion, meningoencephalitis, facial palsy, peripheral neuropathy, dorsal root ganglionitis (acute ataxic neuropathy), transverse myelitis, and polymyositis. Chronic neurological problems include vacuolar myelopathy, peripheral neuropathy, and AIDS dementia complex. Other infections are also common: cytomegalovirus radiculopathy, cryptococcal meningitis, toxoplasmosis (cerebral abscesses), progressive multifocal leucoencephalopathy (PML), and tuberculous meningitis and atypical mycobacteria. In addition, tumours such as primary central nervous system B cell lymphoma may occur

METABOLIC AND TOXIC NEUROPATHIES

Diabetes mellitus

Diabetes is the commonest cause of neuropathy in the UK. It may cause symptoms and signs, or symptoms without signs, or may be asymptomatic. It is more common with poorly controlled diabetics and may occur with insulin-dependant (IDDM) or non-insulin-dependant (NIDDM) diabetes mellitus. The pathological cause remains uncertain (possibly microangiopathy or glycosylation of nerves). The neuropathy is usually axonal. To some extent, the problems are preventable and may be improved by good diabetic control. There are four main clinical patterns of neuropathy:

- Symmetrical sensory peripheral neuropathy: most common, causing numbness, pain, and tingling, usually in the feet, sometimes with weakness (a sensorimotor neuropathy). If severe, a neuropathic (Charcot) joint may result, with painless destruction and disorganization of the joint.
- Autonomic neuropathy: may affect the genitourinary system (with impotence and bladder problems), sweating (e.g. gustatory sweating—facial sweating stimulated by eating), the gastrointestinal tract (with gastric atony, nocturnal diarrhoea, constipation), the cardiovascular system (especially with postural hypotension).
- Isolated nerve lesions (mononeuropathy): especially cranial nerve III (notably sparing the pupil) and at the more common sites of nerve compression in the limbs. Diabetic amyotrophy is painful wasting and weakness in the thigh with a depressed or absent knee jerk which may be caused by a femoral nerve neuropathy.
- Multiple mononeuropathy (affecting more than one nerve, but sparing others) (see Hint and Tip, p. 213)

Careful monitoring of diabetic patients for early signs of neuropathy is therefore essential.

Causes of a neuropathic (Charcot) joint:
- **Diabetes mellitus**
- **Syringomyelia**
- **Syphilis (tabes dorsalis)**
- **Hereditary sensory neuropathy**
- **Leprosy**

Other metabolic and endocrine causes

Metabolic causes of neuropathy include:
- Vitamin B_{12} deficiency.
- Alcohol (possibly caused by direct toxicity or thiamine deficiency).
- Thiamine deficiency (beriberi).
- Pyridoxine deficiency (e.g. with isoniazid therapy).
- Severe chronic renal failure.
- Chronic, severe vitamin E deficiency.
- Liver failure (rare).

Endocrine causes include:
- Thyrotoxicosis.
- Myxoedema.
- Acromegaly.

Toxic neuropathies

Drugs:
- Antibiotics: isoniazid, nitrofurantoin, metronidazole.
- Chemotherapeutic agents: vincristine, cisplatin.
- Psychotherapeutic agents: lithium, tricyclic antidepressants.

Industrial agents:
- Organic solvents (e.g. *n*-hexane, may affect glue-sniffers), acrylamide.
- Toluene.
- Arsenic (insecticides).
- Organophosphorus agents.
- Lead (contamination of drinking water from old pipes).
- Thallium (pesticides).
- Triorthocresyl phosphate (high-temperature lubricant).

Neurological features of B_{12} deficiency:
- **Sensory neuropathy (common)**
- **Dorsal column sensory loss**
- **Subacute combined degeneration of the cord (dorsal column plus corticospinal loss)**
- **Dementia**
- **Depression**
- **Optic atrophy**

vessels) and is associated with a rash. In adults, but not in children, it may be associated with underlying malignancy (in 20% of those over 50 years).

Both conditions respond to steroids.

Inclusion body myositis

This condition is more common in the elderly, especially in men. Features include progressive distal and proximal weakness. It does not respond to steroids.

Polymyalgia rheumatica

This is an important disorder in the elderly with an incidence of 100/100 000 over the age of 50 years. It is

Classification of muscle/neuromuscular junction disorders	
Type of disorder	**Examples**
muscular dystrophy	Duchenne's, Becker's, facioscapulohumeral, limb-girdle, myotonic dystrophy
inflammatory myopathy	polymyositis, dermatomyositis, inclusion body myositis, infective myositis, polymyalgia rheumatica
metabolic myopathy	McArdles's disease, mitochondrial disorders, periodic paralyses
endocrine myopathy	thyroid disease, Cushing's disease
drug-induced myopathy	clofibrate, D-penicillamine, steroids, alcohol
disorders of neuromuscular transmission	myasthenia gravis, Lambert–Eaton myasthenic syndrome, stiff-man syndrome

Fig. 15.4 Classification of muscle/neuromuscular junction disorders.

The periodic paralyses	
Hyperkalaemic periodic paralysis	**Hypokalaemic periodic paralysis**
sodium-channel mutations, chromosome 17	calcium-channel mutations, chromosome 1
autosomal recessive	autosomal dominant
occurs with rest after exercise and may have periocular myotonia	occurs after meals and with rest after exercise
short attacks of weakness (about 1 hour) which may be aborted by exercise at onset	weakness for several hours

Fig. 15.5 The potassium channel periodic paralyses. Note, however, that the presentations are often identical, and the conditions cannot often be differentiated clinically.

ssociated with cranial arteritis and importantly, there is a risk of sudden blindness if it is untreated. The condition is sensitive to steroids.

Metabolic myopathies

All metabolic myopathies are rare. McArdle's disease, a glycogenosis caused by deficiency of myophosphorylase, is one of many such disorders, and is associated with painful muscle cramps and weakness after exercise. Recently, the periodic paralyses (see Fig. 15.5) have been found to be caused by ion-channel mutations and are now included in the class of disorders know as 'channelopathies'.

Disorders of neuromuscular transmission

Myasthenia gravis

The prevalence of myasthenia gravis is about 5/100 000. Women are affected twice as frequently as men. The condition is characterized by fatiguable weakness of periocular, facial, and proximal muscles, i.e. it worsens with exercise, and usually gets worse as the day goes on (diurnal).

Myasthenia gravis is associated with acetylcholine-receptor antibodies. Both immunologic and genetic factors seem important in its pathogenesis.

The condition is associated with lymphoid hyperplasia and tumours of the thymus, and weakness may respond to surgical removal of this, especially in young patients with a short history. Otherwise, treatment is with immunosuppression and with anticholinesterases.

Lambert–Eaton myasthenic syndrome

This is characterized by weakness that is initially lessened with exercise. It is a rare disorder, more common in men, and about one-half of cases are associated with an underlying tumour.

- **Describe the types of pathology of muscle that can cause weakness.**
- **What are the characteristics of disorders of the neuromuscular junction?**

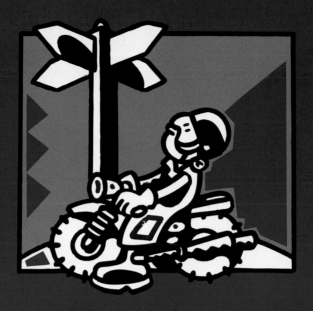

SELF-ASSESSMENT

Multiple-choice Questions

Indicate whether each answer is true or false.

1. A patient is brought into an Accident and Emergency Department unconscious and with neck stiffness.

(a) Lumbar puncture should be performed immediately.
(b) A purpuric rash is most suggestive of pneumococcal meningitis.
(c) Subarachnoid haemorrhage may be the underlying cause.
(d) Intracranial tumour is ruled out by neck stiffness.
(e) The patient should be observed for 30 minutes to see if helpful focal signs develop.

2. In the eye:

(a) The cornea has no sensory innervation.
(b) Ganglion cell axons are unmyelinated inside the eye.
(c) The sclera is continuous with the arachnoid layer.
(d) The fovea contains only rods.
(e) Branches of the central retinal artery do not pass over the fovea.

3. Regarding dementia:

(a) Patients with Pick's disease have a cortical dementia.
(b) Dementia is a rare clinical feature of Parkinson's disease.
(c) A mini-mental state score of 28 is suggestive of dementia, provided that the patient is not depressed or in an acute confusional state.
(d) EEG is very helpful in making the diagnosis.
(e) Alzheimer's disease is the cause of dementia in about 40% of cases.

4. Concerning anxiolytics and anticonvulsants:

(a) Benzodiazepines block GABA action by binding to the GABA receptor.
(b) Benzodiazepine action can be prolonged by active metabolites.
(c) Intravenous clonazepam is used to treat status epilepticus.
(d) Phenytoin action shows a use dependency.
(e) Valproate has only one mechanism of action similar to phenytoin.

5. In cerebrovascular disease:

(a) Total anterior circulation infarction (TACI) has a high early mortality and recurrence rate.
(b) Lacunar infarctions can present with isolated dysphasia.
(c) Subarachnoid haemorrhage is usually caused by a rupture of a Charcot–Bouchard aneurysm.
(d) Lateral medullary syndrome is caused by acute occlusion of the posterior inferior cerebellar artery.
(e) Amaurosis fugax is suggestive of a contralateral carotid lesion.

6. A young man presents who, over the past 2 days, has developed weakness in his hands and feet. Since this morning he has been unable to stand up and cannot lift his arms above his head.

(a) He may have a lumbosacral disc protrusion.
(b) A complaint of numb toes makes Guillain–Barré syndrome less likely.
(c) Increased reflexes and extensor plantar responses indicate a probable intracranial problem.
(d) A history of recent diarrhoea is unlikely to be important.
(e) Peak expiratory flow rate should be monitored.

7. Concerning taste and smell:

(a) Fungiform papillae are found on the anterior two-thirds of the tongue.
(b) The olfactory epithelium sends projections to the olfactory bulb.
(c) Taste afferents synapse in the solitary nucleus.
(d) Granule cells in the olfactory bulb project into the cortex.
(e) Afferents to the olfactory cortex synapse first in the thalamus.

8. In a 55-year-old woman with a brain tumour:

(a) In the presence of a dressing apraxia, the lesion is likely to be in the dominant parietal lobe.
(b) The presence of upper quadrant homonymous field defect suggests that the lesion is likely to be in the temporal lobe.
(c) Sensory inattention is suggestive of a dominant hemispheric lesion.
(d) Altered personality and loss of initiative suggests that the lesion is likely to be in the frontal lobe.
(e) The presence of dyscalculia suggests a temporal lobe lesion.

9. A 60-year-old woman presents to an Accident and Emergency Department. She was found in the street 30 minutes previously and has been fitting since.

(a) CT brain scan is the first priority.
(b) She may respond to intravenous diazepam.
(c) If the fitting stops she can be discharged.
(d) The diagnosis is status epilepticus. Further investigation is not necessary.
(e) If the seizure continues, she should be transferred to a neurosurgical centre.

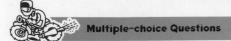

10. Concerning memory and the limbic system:

(a) Lesions of the hippocampus and surrounding area can produce amnesia.
(b) The parahippocampal gyrus is continuous with the cingulate gyrus.
(c) Primacy effects are caused by long-term memory.
(d) Procedural memory can be spared in amnesia.
(e) Working memory has a capacity of 7±2 units of information.

11. A 54-year-old patient presents with diplopia.

(a) The presence of ptosis, and divergent squint is suggestive of a lesion of cranial nerve III.
(b) If diplopia is present when reading or looking down, then a lesion of cranial nerve VI is likely.
(c) The pupil is likely to be spared in diabetic lesions of cranial nerve III.
(d) Fluctuating diplopia is suggestive of myasthenia gravis.
(e) If caused by an acute palsy of cranial nerve III, and associated with an acute severe headache and signs of meningism, then a posterior communicating artery aneurysm should be excluded.

12. Concerning nystagmus:

(a) Nystagmus is jerky, with the fast phase to the side of the lesion in unilateral vestibular lesions.
(b) Downbeating nystagmus is suggestive of a lesion at or around the superior colliculi.
(c) Pendular nystagmus is suggestive of long-standing impaired macular vision.
(d) Nystagmus is suggestive of a brainstem pathology if its direction varies with the direction of gaze.
(e) Nystagmus is often symptomatic.

13. A 66-year-old patient presents with lower cranial nerve palsies.

(a) A wasted and fasciculation tongue is suggestive of pseudobulbar palsy.
(b) The jaw jerk is brisk in pseudobulbar palsy, but absent in bulbar palsy.
(c) Motor neuron disease causes features of both bulbar and pseudobulbar palsy.
(d) Speech is monotonous in bulbar palsy.
(e) Emotional lability is suggestive of pseudobulbar palsy.

14. A 19-year-old man is referred by the orthopaedic surgeons before surgery for bilateral pes cavus.

(a) Spina bifida may be the cause.
(b) A chronic peripheral neuropathy, such as is seen with diabetes mellitus may, cause this picture.
(c) This could be caused by porphyria.
(d) The condition has probably developed in the past year.
(e) Nerve conduction studies may be abnormal.

15. In the brain:

(a) The internal capsule is lateral to the lentiform nucleus.
(b) The amygdala lies in the frontal lobe.
(c) The frontal lobe is separated from the parietal lobe by the precentral sulcus.
(d) The hippocampus lies in the temporal lobe.
(e) The lateral sulcus lies between the parietal lobe and the occipital lobe.

16. In the development of the central nervous system:

(a) Cells of the neural tube form dorsal root ganglion cells.
(b) Cells of the neural tube form glia and neurons.
(c) The brain develops from three vesicles.
(d) Failure of neural tube closure can result in spinal and cranial defects.
(e) Basal plate cells develop into cells with sensory function.

17. Regarding brain tumours:

(a) Glioblastoma multiformis is a tumour of childhood.
(b) Meningioma is the commonest benign primary brain tumour.
(c) CT scanning is the preferred method of investigating tumours of the pituitary fossa because, unlike MRI, the images will not be affected by artefacts from the surrounding bony structures.
(d) Calcified tumours are always benign.
(e) Bronchogenic carcinoma is the commonest primary systemic tumour in metastatic brain tumours.

18. Concerning the action potential:

(a) IPSPs are caused by increasing membrane permeability to cations, e.g. Na^+.
(b) Temporal summation occurs only when there is transmission at many synapses.
(c) There are few Na^+ channels at the axon hillock.
(d) Conduction velocity (m/s) in myelinated axons is six times the diameter (μm).
(e) After demyelination, axonal membranes can store more charge.

19. Concerning the spinal cord:

(a) The spinothalamic tract carries ipsilateral sensory information.
(b) The dorsal columns carry ipsilateral sensory information.
(c) The lateral corticospinal tract carries crossed fibres.
(d) The tectospinal tract carries information to the midbrain.
(e) Dorsal column axons are thicker than spinothalamic axons.

20. Cerebral oedema.

(a) Vasogenic oedema is an intracellular oedema.
(b) Cytotoxic oedema affects both grey and white matter.
(c) Vasogenic oedema is usually responsive to treatment with steroids, mannitol, and dehydration.
(d) Hydrocephalus may result in extracellular oedema.
(e) Hypoxic brain damage usually results in cytotoxic oedema.

21. Concerning pain:

(a) Nociceptors have unencapsulated endings.
(b) Local circuits in the dorsal horn influence pain signal transmission.
(c) Opioids act only in the dorsal horn.
(d) In morphine overdose the pupils are dilated.
(e) Naloxone is an antagonist at the µ receptor.

22. At the synapse:

(a) Neurotransmitters are released at all synapses.
(b) Axoaxonic synapses can inhibit action potential generation.
(c) Intracellular Na^+ is the signal for exocytosis.
(d) Dopamine synthesis is regulated by altering the activity of dopa decarboxylase.
(e) Neurotransmission can be terminated by uptake into the terminal bouton.

23. Concerning the pyramidal tract:

(a) The pyramidal tract contains only axons originating in the primary motor cortex.
(b) The pyramidal tract passes through the posterior one-third of the internal capsule.
(c) The motor homunculus has large hands.
(d) Upper motor neuron lesions result in atrophy and fasciculation.
(e) The lateral corticospinal tract innervates distal limb muscles.

24. Concerning dysphasia:

(a) Lesions of the angular gyrus cause a non-fluent dysphasia.
(b) Repetition is impaired in conductive dysphasia.
(c) Lesions at Broca's area cause fluent dysphasia.
(d) Dysphasias are caused by non-dominant hemispheric lesions.
(e) Cerebrovascular disease and brain tumours are the commonest causes of dysphasia.

25. Concerning basal ganglia:

(a) The striatum has poor connections with the cortex.
(b) The substantia nigra sends a dopaminergic projection to the striatum.
(c) The indirect processing loop via the subthalamic nucleus excites the cortex.
(d) L-Dopa is given to Parkinsonian patients because it is metabolized by tyrosine hydroxylase.
(e) The basal ganglia are involved in the activation of motor programs.

26. Parkinson's disease:

(a) Is always an obvious diagnosis.
(b) Should be treated immediately with L-dopa.
(c) Is an upper motor neuron disorder, and therefore associated with increased tendon reflexes.
(d) Symptoms may respond to anticholinergic drugs.
(e) Is associated with depression.

27. In the cerebellum:

(a) Mossy fibres carry proprioceptive information.
(b) Purkinje cells send excitatory projections to the deep cerebellar nuclei.
(c) Cerebellar hemispheres process ipsilateral motor functions.
(d) Cerebellar lesions produce ataxia.
(e) Complex spikes recorded in granule cells signal error detection.

28. In the autonomic nervous system:

(a) Preganglionic fibres are unmyelinated.
(b) All parasympathetic preganglionic neurons have their cell bodies in the brainstem.
(c) Muscarinic antagonists reduce heart rate.
(d) Acetylcholine is released at all ganglia.
(e) One preganglionic sympathetic neuron can synapse in several ganglia.

29. Concerning the auditory system:

(a) The basilar membrane is of uniform width.
(b) Hair cells show different frequency sensitivities along the basilar membrane.
(c) Feedback from the brainstem travels in the olivocochlear bundle.
(d) Pathways from the cochlear nuclei travel only contralaterally up to the cortex.
(e) The primary auditory cortex is in the parietal lobe.

30. Concerning somatosensation:

(a) Rapidly adapting receptors continue firing while their stimulus is still present.
(b) Axons from proprioceptors are unmyelinated.
(c) The cell bodies of spinothalamic tract axons lie in dorsal root ganglia.
(d) The sensory homunculus has very small hands.
(e) The sensory cortex lies in the parietal lobe.

31. Concerning the localization of cortical function:

(a) The cerebral hemispheres have similar processing functions.
(b) Frontal lobe lesions can result in disorders of object recognition.
(c) Planning deficits can result from frontal lobe lesions.
(d) Lesions to the motor cortex supplying the laryngeal muscles lead to copious production of nonsense sounds.
(e) Parietal lobe lesions can produce attentional disorders.

32. Concerning cognitive development and degeneration:

(a) The newborn child has no cognitive abilities.
(b) The sensorimotor stage is the first in Piaget's scheme of development.
(c) Successful ageing occurs without relative synaptogenesis.
(d) Small cell numbers in the cortex increase with age.
(e) Social withdrawal in the elderly cannot be reversed.

33. Concerning central visual pathways:

(a) Fibres from the nasal half of the retina cross over in the chiasm.
(b) There are cells in the lateral geniculate nucleus that receive information from both eyes.
(c) Lesions of the optic tract affect both sides of the visual field.
(d) The primary visual cortex has a columnar organization.
(e) Most of the visual cortex is devoted to processing the peripheral visual field.

34. Concerning antidepressants and antipsychotics:

(a) The cheese reaction occurs because of inhibition of cerebral monoamine oxidase by monoamine oxidase inhibitors.
(b) Tricyclics show an antimuscarinic and antiadrenergic side-effect profile.
(c) Antipsychotic potency is proportional to D_4 blocking ability.
(d) The motor side effects of antipsychotics are due to effects on the pyramidal system.
(e) Clozapine blocks the D_2 receptor preferentially.

35. Regarding developmental and associated disorders:

(a) Children with cerebral palsy have mental retardation.
(b) A patient in whom spina bifida is picked up on an incidental radiograph should be referred for a surgical opinion to prevent later deterioration.
(c) Hydrocephalus is diagnosed by ultrasonography in adults and children.
(d) Dementia with normal-pressure hydrocephalus may respond to surgery.
(e) Arnold–Chiari formation may cause headache.

36. Concerning brainstem-acting drugs:

(a) 5-HT_3 antagonists act only at the chemoreceptor trigger zone.
(b) Antihistamines reduce nausea caused by vestibular input to the vomiting centre.
(c) Dopamine agonists reduce nausea.
(d) The potency of an inhaled general anaesthetic agent is related to its blood:gas coefficient.
(e) General anaesthetic agents produce cardiovascular depression.

37. In a patient with bilateral wasting and weakness of the small hand muscles:

(a) The findings are explicable in terms of bilateral cerebral lesions.
(b) The findings could be caused by rheumatoid arthritis.
(c) Absence of the biceps jerk excludes cervical spondylosis as a cause.
(d) Extensor plantar responses exclude cervical spondylosis as a cause.
(e) Syringomyelia is one of the commonest causes.

38. Following one epileptic seizure in an adult:

(a) Driving is allowed but must stop if a second event occurs.
(b) A brain scan should be performed in most cases.
(c) Lumbar puncture is mandatory.
(d) EEG showing three-per-second spike-and-wave activity indicates a likely structural lesion.
(e) The probability of a second event within 3 years is 50%.

39. A 25-year-old man presented to and Accident and Emergency Department with a head injury.

(a) Skull radiography is essential.
(b) The risk of chronic subdural haematoma is related to the severity of the head injury.
(c) He is said to have had a concussion if only minor macroscopic brain damage has occurred.
(d) Extradural haematoma is usually caused by a rupture of the sagittal or transverse sinuses.
(e) The risk of post-traumatic epilepsy is increased if he develops an epileptic seizure in the first 24 hours after injury.

40. EEG:

(a) Is necessary for the diagnosis of brain death.
(b) May be used in the diagnosis of metabolic encephalopathy.
(c) If normal, makes epilepsy unlikely.
(d) Is normal following a stroke.
(e) May be abnormal in migraine.

41. In the motor unit:

(a) Large innervation ratios give fine control over movement.
(b) Smaller motor neurons are recruited before larger ones.
(c) Fast fibres contain glycolytic enzymes.
(d) Fibre clumping occurs with diseases of the muscle fibres.
(e) Spontaneous muscle activity can occur in diseases of the motor neuron.

42. Regarding numbness in the leg:

(a) A numb patch on the lateral surface of the thigh is often of ominous cause.
(b) Numbness on the sole of the foot should be associated with an absent knee jerk.
(c) If associated with a rash, may be caused by shingles.
(d) Bilateral proximal numbness is associated with diabetes mellitus.
(e) Is a recognized feature of motor neuron disease.

43. Concerning the brainstem:

(a) The pyramidal tracts decussate at the top of the medulla.
(b) The trigeminal nucleus receives somatosensory information from cranial nerves other than the trigeminal.
(c) Cranial nerve X leaves the medulla lateral to the olivary nucleus.
(d) The nuclei of cranial nerves VI and VII are closely related.
(e) Cranial nerve III emerges between the cerebral peduncles.

44. Winging of the scapula:

(a) Is seen in some forms of muscular dystrophy.
(b) May be neurogenic or myogenic.
(c) Is caused by a lesion of the nerve to subscapularis.
(d) Usually recovers completely.
(e) Causes difficulty lifting the arm on that side.

45. In the ventricles:

(a) Cerebrospinal fluid is secreted by the choroid plexus.
(b) Blockage of the aqueduct causes a communicating hydrocephalus.
(c) The lateral ventricles drain directly into the fourth ventricle.
(d) The ventricular cavities are lined with pia mater.
(e) Cerebrospinal fluid has the same protein content as plasma.

46. A 60-year-old man has a 5-year history of dizziness and sometimes faints when he stands up quickly.

(a) This sounds like epilepsy.
(b) A carotid bruit might be significant.
(c) If he also has impotence, unsteadiness, and slurred speech, this could fit with multiple system atrophy.
(d) A drop of systolic blood pressure of 40 mmHg on standing might be incidental.
(e) The symptoms could be caused by cardiac disease.

47. In central nervous system infections:

(a) *Neisseria meningitidis, Streptococcus pneumoniae,* and *Haemophilus influenzae* are the commonest causative organisms of epidural spinal abscesses.
(b) Viral meningitis is a benign and self-limiting disease and no specific treatment is required.
(c) In meningitis, lumbar puncture should always be performed before initiating antibiotic treatment.
(d) Acyclovir is nephrotoxic and should be used only in confirmed cases of herpes simplex encephalitis.
(e) Toxoplasmosis is a common fungal infection in AIDS patients.

48. Concerning the vestibular system:

(a) The otolith organs detect head position.
(b) The vestibulospinal tracts influence antigravity muscles.
(c) The vestibular nuclei project to cranial nerve nuclei controlling eye position.
(d) The horizontal vestibulo-ocular reflex uses complementary information from both cranial nerves VIII.
(e) Proprioception is mediated only by sensations from the musculoskeletal system.

49. Regarding metabolic and toxic diseases of the nervous system:

(a) Thiamine deficiency may result in neuropathy, dementia, or myelopathy (subacute combined degeneration of the cord).
(b) Abrupt alcohol withdrawal may result in delirium tremens which presents with tremor, hallucinations, seizures, and autonomic overactivity.
(c) Lead poisoning causes chronic painful sensory neuropathy.
(d) Confusion, ataxia, and oculomotor disturbances are early features of Wernicke–Korsakoff syndrome.
(e) Carbon monoxide poisoning causes chronic encephalopathy with ataxia, dysarthria, and tremor.

50. Myotonic dystrophy:

(a) Is caused by the same sort of molecular abnormality as Friedreich's ataxia.
(b) Is a particular type of Duchenne's muscular dystrophy.
(c) Is associated with cardiac arrhythmias.
(d) Is inherited through either parent.
(e) Is associated with sustained muscle contractions.

Short-answer Questions

1. Draw a cross-section through the spinal cord. Label the sensory tracts with the type of sensory information they carry.

2. A previously fit 25-year-old patient comes to outpatients with a short history of vertigo precipitated by head movements. Hallpike's manoeuvre was found to be positive.
   (a) How is Hallpike's manoeuvre done?
   (b) What are the clinical features of central and peripheral positional vertigo?

3. (a) What are the causes of tremor in a 60-year-old man?
   (b) Outline the features you would look for on examination to aid your diagnosis.

4. Why do parasympathetic signals reach their target organs more quickly than sympathetic signals?

5. A patient presents with the typical features of Guillain–Barré syndrome
   (a) What are these?
   (b) What other diagnoses would you consider?

6. A 44-year-old woman presents with a traumatic cervical spinal injury following a road traffic accident. On examination she is found to have paraparesis.
   (a) What are the possible pathological processes responsible for her neurological deficit?
   (b) Outline the management of this patient.

7. With a series of diagrams, describe the process of neurulation. What can happen if the neural tube fails to close?

8. (a) What are the three types of hydrocephalus?
   (b) Outline the clinical features of hydrocephalus briefly.

9. List the functions of glial cells.

10. A 38-year-old woman comes to outpatients with a history of two episodes of 'feeling funny' with an odd sensation in her right arm, followed by loss of consciousness.
    (a) What is the most likely diagnosis and how would you confirm this?
    (b) How would you treat the patient?

11. What does the jacksonian march tell us about the organisation of the motor cortex?

12. Name two drugs that act on the brainstem to reduce vomiting and describe their different mechanisms of action.

13. With the aid of a diagram, show the activation cascade for light signal transduction in the photoreceptor.

14. A 60-year-old woman has tingling in her middle and index fingers, especially troublesome at night.
    (a) What is the most common cause of these symptoms?
    (b) What would you particularly look for in the history and examination?

15. A 32-year-old man complains that he has difficulty walking upstairs and getting up from a chair.
    (a) Where would you expect to find muscle weakness?
    (b) What are the possible diagnoses?

16. How do the contents of the middle ear transmit and amplify sound?

17. A 21-year-old woman with multiple sclerosis was admitted to hospital following a relapse.
    (a) Describe the possible clinical features of multiple sclerosis.
    (b) What investigations would have been used to confirm the diagnosis in this patient.?

18. Why do we have loss of taste with a blocked-up nose?

19. Describe how we can distinguish between working memory and long-term memory.

20. A 55-year-old woman presents to outpatients with a one-year history of difficulty in walking. On examination she was found to be ataxic.
    (a) Outline the clinical features of ataxic gait.
    (b) How do you differentiate clinically between the two types of ataxic gait?

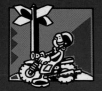
1. Describe in outline how the various parts of the motor system contribute to motor processing.

2. A young man arrives in an Accident and Emergency Department at midnight when you are the house officer on duty. He is unconscious but breathing spontaneously. He is unaccompanied. Describe your management.

3. Discuss general medical disorders that may be associated with numbness of the hands and feet.

4. Discuss the clinical features of speech disorders.

5. What are the consequences of different types of damage to peripheral axons?

6. The mental state examination is an essential part of the neurological assessment. Discuss its different components.

7. Discuss the risk factors, the pathological mechanisms, and the clinical features of stroke.

8. Describe the mechanism of opioid analgesia. What are the dangers of opioid overdose and how can they be treated?

9. Give an account of the central visual pathways with examples of how lesions can affect the visual field.

10. Give an account of the drug treatment of depression. Do you believe the monoamine theory?

MCQ Answers

1. (a) F, (b) F, (c) T, (d) F, (e) F
2. (a) F, (b) T, (c) F, (d) F, (e) T
3. (a) T, (b) F, (c) F, (d) F, (e) F
4. (a) F, (b) T, (c) T, (d) T, (e) F
5. (a) F, (b) F, (c) F, (d) T, (e) F
6. (a) F, (b) F, (c) F, (d) F, (e) F
7. (a) T, (b) T, (c) T, (d) F, (e) F
8. (a) F, (b) T, (c) F, (d) T, (e) F
9. (a) F, (b) T, (c) F, (d) F, (e) F
10. (a) T, (b) T, (c) T, (d) T, (e) T
11. (a) T, (b) F, (c) T, (d) T, (e) T
12. (a) F, (b) F, (c) T, (d) T, (e) F
13. (a) F, (b) F, (c) T, (d) F, (e) T
14. (a) T, (b) F, (c) F, (d) F, (e) T
15. (a) F, (b) F, (c) F, (d) T, (e) F
16. (a) F, (b) T, (c) T, (d) T, (e) F
17. (a) F, (b) T, (c) F, (d) F, (e) T
18. (a) F, (b) F, (c) F, (d) T, (e) T
19. (a) F, (b) T, (c) T, (d) F, (e) T
20. (a) F, (b) T, (c) T, (d) T, (e) T
21. (a) T, (b) T, (c) F, (d) F, (e) T
22. (a) F, (b) T, (c) F, (d) F, (e) T
23. (a) F, (b) T, (c) T, (d) F, (e) T
24. (a) F, (b) T, (c) F, (d) F, (e) T
25. (a) F, (b) T, (c) F, (d) F, (e) T

26. (a) F, (b) F, (c) F, (d) T, (e) T
27. (a) T, (b) F, (c) T, (d) T, (e) F
28. (a) F, (b) F, (c) F, (d) T, (e) T
29. (a) F, (b) T, (c) T, (d) F, (e) F
30. (a) F, (b) F, (c) F, (d) F, (e) T
31. (a) F, (b) F, (c) T, (d) F, (e) T
32. (a) F, (b) T, (c) F, (d) T, (e) F
33. (a) T, (b) F, (c) F, (d) T, (e) F
34. (a) F, (b) T, (c) F, (d) F, (e) F
35. (a) F, (b) F, (c) F, (d) T, (e) T
36. (a) F, (b) T, (c) F, (d) F, (e) T
37. (a) F, (b) T, (c) F, (d) F, (e) F
38. (a) F, (b) T, (c) F, (d) F, (e) T
39. (a) F, (b) F, (c) F, (d) F, (e) T
40. (a) F, (b) T, (c) F, (d) F, (e) T
41. (a) F, (b) T, (c) T, (d) F, (e) T
42. (a) F, (b) F, (c) T, (d) F, (e) F
43. (a) F, (b) T, (c) T, (d) T, (e) T
44. (a) T, (b) T, (c) F, (d) F, (e) T
45. (a) T, (b) F, (c) F, (d) F, (e) F
46. (a) F, (b) T, (c) T, (d) F, (e) T
47. (a) F, (b) T, (c) F, (d) F, (e) F
48. (a) T, (b) T, (c) T, (d) T, (e) F
49. (a) F, (b) T, (c) F, (d) T, (e) F
50. (a) T, (b) F, (c) T, (d) T, (e) T

SAQ Answers

1. See Figs 3.9 and 3.13. Dorsal columns labelled with ipsilateral proprioceptive and fine touch information. Spinothalamic tract labelled with contralateral crude touch, pain, and temperature information.

2. (a) Briefly describe how to perform this manoeuvre.
(b) Positive Hallpike's manoeuvre can be due to a peripheral (semicircular canals) or central (brainstem) pathology (Fig. 12.25).

3. (a) (i) Part of a general illness; for example, thyrotoxicosis, alcohol dependence, hepatic failure.
(ii) Owing to neurological disease, e.g. action tremor (drugs, essential), resting (parkinsonism), intention (cerebellar). Confused with tremor, e.g. pseudoathetosis.
(b) Note: the question asked for examination, not history. (i) General, e.g. tachycardia, goitre, hepatomegaly
(ii) Specific, e.g. at rest, on action only, with intention, with eyes shut (pseudoathetosis), bradykinesia, rigidity, etc. is there a disturbance of eye movement?

4. Preganglionic fibres are myelinated and postganglionic fibres are unmyelinated. In the parasympathetic nervous system the ganglia are close to their target organs, which means that most of the journey from the central nervous system to the target is along myelinated fibres. In the sympathetic nervous system the ganglia are nearer to the cord, e.g. paravertebral chain and mesenteric ganglia. A greater fraction of the signal pathway in the sympathetic nervous system uses unmyelinated fibres.

5. (a) Days–weeks progressive, flaccid, hyporeflexic weakness usually following a gastrointestinal or respiratory illness
(b) See Chapter 15, p. 213.

6. (a) Neurological damage may result from oedema, haemorrhage, compression of the cord by fractured or misaligned vertebrae, or transection of the cord by elements of the vertebral column.
(b) The principles of management include immobilization to prevent further neural damage, preservation of skin integrity, preservation of bladder and bowel function, management of complications (respiratory, cardiovascular, gastrointestinal), and long-term rehabilitation.

7. Fig. 1.2. Neural tube defects can result in malformations of the vertebral column and skull. In the spine these range from defects in the vertebral arch to complete exposure of the spinal cord. In the skull, failure of cranial neuropore closure can result in anencephaly, but less-severe malformations result in defects in the occipital bone.

8. (a) Obstructive, communicating, and compensatory hydrocephalus. Expand.
(b) Clinical features depend on the age of the patient and on whether the hydrocephalus is acute or chronic (Fig. 14.6).

9. Astrocytes—support, nutrition, regulation of extracellular ion concentration, absorption of neurotransmitters, scar formation.
Oligodendrocytes—myelination of central nervous system axons.
Microglia—phagocytosis and antigen presentation.

10. (a) Epilepsy. History—from a witness, and from the patient (how exactly did she feel 'funny'? was she confused on waking? etc.). Examination—since episodes sound like focal seizures with secondary generalization, there may (but often are not) be focal signs.
(b) Explain. Investigate (EEG, CT). Therapy. Advice (driving and avoid precipitants).

11. The jacksonian march is a seizure affecting the motor cortex, producing muscle movement that spreads over the body. As the disordered neuronal firing moves along the motor cortex, it produces action in different muscle groups, which implies that muscles within a group are represented in the same area of the cortex. The fact that movement spreads over the body indicates that the whole body is represented in the cortex in an orderly fashion. This is further evidence for the homuncular organization of the motor cortex.

12. Refer to Fig. 5.4.

13. Refer to Fig. 7.9.

14. (a) Carpal tunnel syndrome.
(b) History: predisposing factors (e.g. occupation—cleaning windows and scrubbing floors can provoke, arthritis, not pregnancy at this age), relieving factors (shaking), history to suggest another cause?, e.g. neck pains, numb feet. Examination: evidence of median nerve compression, no evidence of generalized neuropathy.

15. (a) Proximally.
(b) Inherited (e.g. Becker's or limb girdle muscular dystrophy, metabolic myopathy, not Duchenne's at this age). Acquired (e.g. polymyositis, myasthenia gravis, endocrine disease, neoplastic).

16. The ossicles transmit vibrations from the tympanic membrane to the oval window. The base plate of the stapes has a much smaller surface area than the tympanic membrane so that pressure changes due to sound waves are amplified in the perilymph by movement of the stapes.

17. (a) The symptoms and signs depend on the anatomical location of the plaques (optic nerve: optic neuritis with reduced visual acuity, central scotoma, afferent pupillary defect and pale optic disc; brainstem: abnormal eye movements, limb ataxia, dysarthria and vertigo; spinal cord: sensory symptoms and signs with occasional sensory levels, spastic weakness, sphincter disturbance). Other features include dementia, euphoria, facial pain, and painful tonic spasms.
(b) Multiple sclerosis is a clinical diagnosis. MRI is the most helpful investigation and is abnormal in almost all cases. Cerebrospinal fluid shows oligoclonal bands in 90% of cases. Evoked potentials may be prolonged.

18. We sense a loss of taste because olfaction contributes much more than taste receptors to our perceived sense of taste. In a blocked-up nose, olfactory stimuli have difficulty reaching the olfactory epithelium in the roof of the nasal cavity and so we rely on the poorer information from taste buds.

19. Primacy and recency effects, amnesic patients with preserved long-term memory and poor working memory, the coding system used for information storage and capacity for information storage.

20. (a) The clinical features of sensory and cerebellar ataxic gaits should be discussed.
(b) Romberg's test would help to differentiate between these two types of ataxia. Expand.

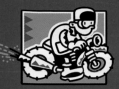

Appendices

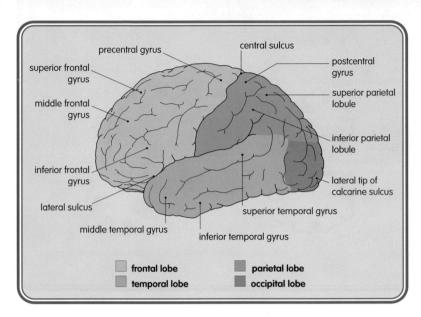

Fig. A1.1 Cerebral hemisphere—lateral view.

precentral gyrus

central sulcus

superior frontal gyrus

postcentral gyrus

middle frontal gyrus

superior parietal lobule

inferior parietal lobule

inferior frontal gyrus

lateral tip of calcarine sulcus

lateral sulcus

middle temporal gyrus

superior temporal gyrus

inferior temporal gyrus

☐ frontal lobe   ☐ parietal lobe
☐ temporal lobe   ☐ occipital lobe

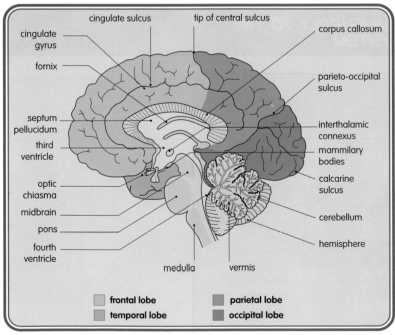

Fig. A1.2 Cerebral hemisphere—medial view.

cingulate sulcus

tip of central sulcus

corpus callosum

cingulate gyrus

fornix

parieto-occipital sulcus

septum pellucidum

interthalamic connexus

third ventricle

mammilary bodies

optic chiasma

calcarine sulcus

midbrain

cerebellum

pons

hemisphere

fourth ventricle

medulla

vermis

☐ frontal lobe   ☐ parietal lobe
☐ temporal lobe   ☐ occipital lobe

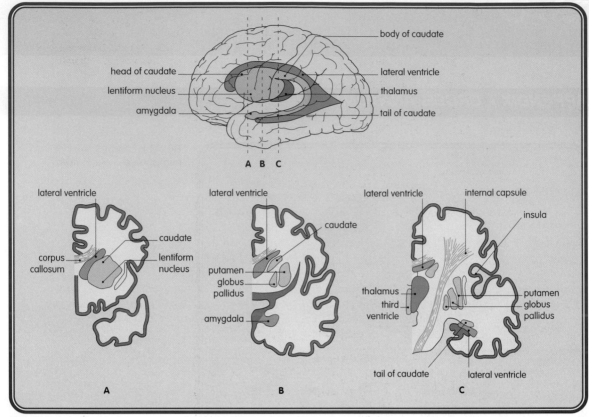

Fig. A1.3 Relationship between basal ganglia, thalamus, and lateral ventricle.

APPENDIX 2. VASCULAR SUPPLY TO THE CENTRAL NERVOUS SYSTEM

Fig. A2.1 Circle of Willis and cranial nerves.

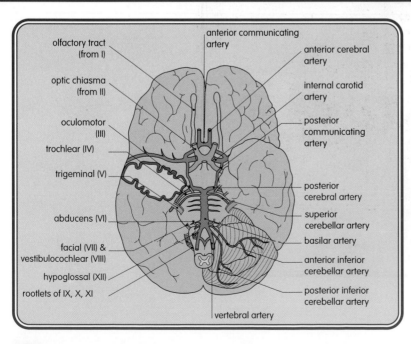

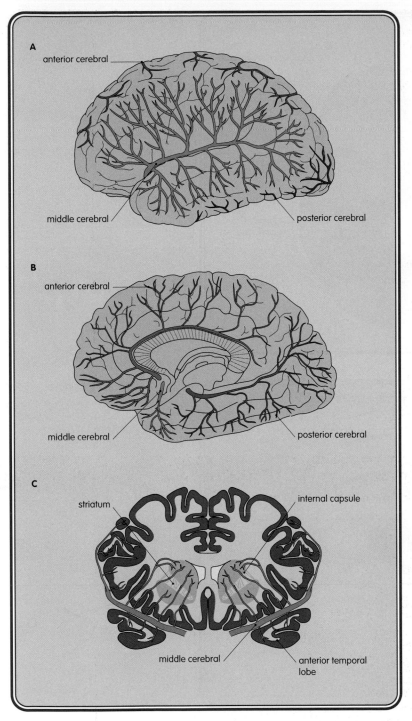

Fig. A2.2 Territories of cerebral arteries. (A) Lateral and (B) medial surfaces of the right cerebral hemispheres. (C) Coronal section of the cerebral hemispheres.

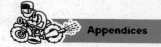

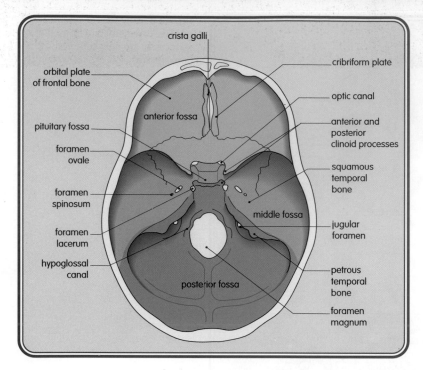

Fig. A2.3 The skull base.

crista galli

orbital plate
of frontal bone

cribriform plate

optic canal

anterior fossa

anterior and
posterior
clinoid processes

pituitary fossa

foramen
ovale

squamous
temporal
bone

foramen
spinosum

middle fossa

jugular
foramen

foramen
lacerum

hypoglossal
canal

posterior fossa

petrous
temporal
bone

foramen
magnum

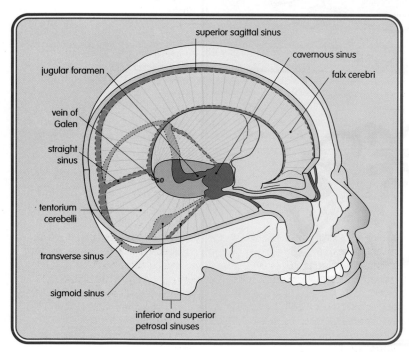

Fig. A2.4 The venous sinuses.

superior sagittal sinus

cavernous sinus

jugular foramen

falx cerebri

vein of
Galen

straight
sinus

tentorium
cerebelli

transverse sinus

sigmoid sinus

inferior and superior
petrosal sinuses

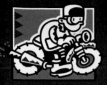

Index

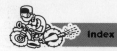

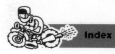

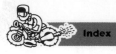

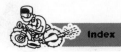

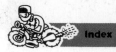